I0438893

The Burden of Digestive Diseases in the United States

JAMES E. EVERHART, M.D., M.P.H., Editor

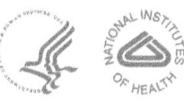

National Institute of Diabetes and Digestive and Kidney Diseases
National Institutes of Health
United States Department of Health and Human Services

COPYRIGHT INFORMATION

All material appearing in this report is in the public domain and may be reproduced or copied without permission: citation as to source, however, is appreciated.

SUGGESTED CITATION

[Author(s). Chapter title. In:] Everhart JE, editor. The burden of digestive diseases in the United States. US Department of Health and Human Services, Public Health Service, National Institutes of Health, National Institute of Diabetes and Digestive and Kidney Diseases. Washington, DC: US Government Printing Office, 2008; NIH Publication No. 09-6443 [pp. –].

Contents

The Burden of Digestive Diseases in the United States

Appendices

Foreword

Digestive diseases include a wide spectrum of disorders affecting the oropharynx and alimentary canal, liver and biliary system, and pancreas. These disorders have diverse causes, including congenital and genetic anomalies, acute and chronic infections, cancer, adverse effects of drugs and toxins, and, in many cases, unknown causes. Some conditions, such as foodborne diarrheal diseases, are so common as to be considered a universal life experience, while many others are relatively uncommon or rare. The impact of these diseases ranges from the inconvenience of a transient diarrheal disease causing missed time from school or work, to chronic and debilitating illnesses requiring continuous medical care, or, all too frequently, to dreaded conditions such as pancreatic cancer that are usually fatal.

During the 20th century, there were dramatic changes in the incidence, prevalence, and overall impact of digestive diseases in the United States that were the result of many factors, including improved sanitation and an improved food supply; numerous research discoveries that led to the development of new drugs, vaccines, diagnostic tests, and minimally invasive procedures; and an economic and health care system capable of providing these advances to the majority of the population. Continued progress in improving the health welfare of the population of the United States requires a continued investment in digestive disease research, public health initiatives, the health care system, and the education of the general public about how to improve their health. Accurate descriptive statistical information is one of the most basic types of information required by those engaged in activities aimed at improving digestive health, including researchers, administrators, public officials, professional and patient-based organizations, and the general public.

In 1994, the National Institutes of Health (NIH) sponsored a publication, *Digestive diseases in the United States: epidemiology and impact*, that has served as a reference to meet these needs; the report had a limited update in 2001.[1,2] Because of continuing changes in the incidence and prevalence of digestive diseases, important changes in health care, such as the emphasis on outpatient care whenever possible, and the availability of new statistical resources, the time is right to generate a new report to capture the impact of digestive diseases in the United States. In addition, congressional report language accompanying the Fiscal Year 2005 appropriations bills in the House and Senate for Labor-Health and Human Services-Education and Related Agencies called for the creation of an advisory committee, the National Commission on Digestive Diseases, and tasked it with addressing the burden of digestive diseases and developing a long-range research plan. The resulting research plan from this charge, *Opportunities and challenges in digestive diseases research: recommendations of the National Commission on Digestive Diseases*, outlines a broad and ambitious agenda aimed at improving the health of the nation for digestive diseases through research; the research plan can be accessed at http://NCDD.niddk. nih.gov. The NIH sponsored the current report on the burden of digestive diseases to serve not only as a needed statistical reference, but also as a companion volume to inform research goals recommended in the Commission's research plan.

Close examination of this report will reveal many interesting and provocative pieces of statistical information about trends in various digestive diseases. As outlined in the report, for any specific disease condition, there are numerous limitations on the types of data that can be obtained in the diverse and decentralized U.S. health care system. Despite the many limitations of the statistical information, there are several certainties. In spite of a century of progress, the burden of digestive diseases in numerical terms remains staggering in the United States; the numbers, however, convey in only a limited way the suffering of and impact on the millions of individuals affected. In addition, the limitations of the report and the statistical data mandate a strong digestive disease research effort aimed at improving health in the United States through pursuit of the many recommendations of the Commission's research plan, improving our ability to capture needed statistical and epidemiological information, and spurring fundamental improvements in the health care system.

Stephen P. James, M.D.
Chair, National Commission on Digestive Diseases
Director, Division of Digestive Diseases and Nutrition
National Institute of Diabetes and Digestive and
 Kidney Diseases
National Institutes of Health
U.S. Department of Health and Human Services

[1] Everhart JE, editor. *Digestive diseases in the United States: epidemiology and impact.* US Department of Health and Human Services, Public Health Service, National Institutes of Health, National Institute of Diabetes and Digestive and Kidney Diseases. Washington, DC: US Government Printing Office, 1994; NIH Publication No. 94-1447.

[2] Sandler RS, Everhart JE, Donowitz M, Adams E, Cronin K, Goodman C, Gemmen E, Shah S, Avdic A, Rubin R. The burden of selected digestive diseases in the United States. *Gastroenterology* 2002;122:1500–1511.

Acknowledgments

I wish to thank the following individuals for making this report possible: Danita Byrd-Holt, Constance Ruhl, Bryan Sayer, Sanee Maphungphong, Beny Wu, Laura Fang, Laura Spofford, Polly Gilbert, Julie Kale, and Katherine Merrell of Social & Scientific Systems, Inc., for programming, production of tables and figures, text and cover graphic design, copyediting, and production of the final report; Daniel Westbrook and Douglas Brown of Georgetown University for analysis of the cost of digestive diseases; David Lieberman and Nora Mattek of the Clinical Outcomes Research Initiative (CORI) for the national endoscopy data; Dedun Ingram at the National Center for Health Statistics for advice on age-adjustment; and Robert Kloos at Ohio State University for advice on recovery times from surgery.

James E. Everhart, M.D., M.P.H., Editor
National Institute of Diabetes and Digestive and Kidney Diseases
National Institutes of Health
U.S. Department of Health and Human Services

CHAPTER 1

All Digestive Diseases

James E. Everhart, M.D., M.P.H.

For systematic coding, mortality and health care statistics rely on disease classification systems, of which the International Classification of Diseases (ICD) is the world standard. The diagnostic codes traditionally used for digestive diseases primarily code for chronic conditions that are neither infectious nor malignant. In the current ICD edition (ICD-10), these include K20 through K93 in chapter "K" (Appendix 1). Other digestive diseases of public health significance and of particular interest to practitioners and researchers are coded in other chapters: Intestinal Infectious and Parasitic Diseases (A00–A09); Viral Hepatitis (B15–B19); Malignant Neoplasms of Digestive Organs (C15–C26); Hemorrhoids (I84); Esophageal and Gastric Varices (I85, I86.4); Maternal Disorders (Digestive) Related to Pregnancy (O21–O22); Conditions (Digestive) Originating in the Perinatal Period (P53, P54, P57, and P59); Digestive System Disorders of Fetus and Newborn (P75–P78, P92); and Congenital Malformations, Deformations, and Chromosomal Abnormalities (Q39–Q45). For some of these groups of conditions, there were enough national data for individual sections in this report. For others, they and many other digestive system disorders were grouped under "other digestive diseases," so that a more complete impact of the total burden of digestive diseases could be estimated.

ICD-9 codes were used for mortality 1979–1998, and ICD-10 codes have been used subsequently, which has been noted on figures of mortality trends. As of the publication of this report, the United States had yet to switch from ICD-9-CM (Clinical Modification) to ICD-10 codes for coding morbidity, despite the publication of the newer edition in 1992. Therefore, all morbidity information from 1979 through 2005 was from ICD-9-CM.

In 2004, there were an estimated 72 million ambulatory care visits with a first-listed diagnosis of a digestive disease and more than 104 million visits with an all-listed diagnoses, which equated to a rate of 35,684

visits per 100,000 U.S. population (Table 1). In other words, for every 100 U.S. residents, there were 35 ambulatory care visits at which a digestive disease diagnosis was noted. Visits were common for all age groups, with the highest rate among persons age 65 years and older. Age-adjusted rates were comparable for blacks and whites and were 20 percent higher for females than for males.

Digestive diseases were common all-listed diagnoses at hospital discharge in 2004 as well as first-listed diagnosis (Table 1). There were approximately 4.6 million discharges of patients with digestive disease as first-listed diagnosis and 13.5 million discharges as all-listed diagnoses. With a rate of all-listed diagnoses of 4,608 per 100,000, there were nearly five overnight hospital stays per 100 U.S. residents that included a discharge diagnosis of at least one digestive disease. These rates were nearly as high among children as among middle-aged adults and were higher in these two age groups than among younger adults. The highest rate was among persons age 65 years and older. In contrast to their ambulatory care visits, blacks had higher rates of hospitalization than did whites. Comparable or lower age-adjusted rates of ambulatory care visits among blacks, yet higher rates of hospitalization, were a common finding for a number of digestive diseases. Women had a 10 percent higher age-adjusted rate than men.

The rate of ambulatory care visits over time (age-adjusted to the 2000 U.S. population) is shown in Figure 1 by 3-year periods (except for the first period, which is 2 years), between 1992 and 2005 (beginning with 1992–1993 and ending with 2003–2005). Age-adjusted rates increased during this period by one-third, from 26.4 per 100 population to 35.3 per 100 population. This trend in increased rates of ambulatory care visits started at least as early as 1985, when there were 22.4 digestive disease diagnoses per 100 population.[1] Rates of all-listed hospitalization with a digestive disease diagnosis fell between 1983 and

1988, a pattern that occurred for all hospitalizations in the United States. Hospitalization rates were stable for the next 10 years before rising to a rate in 2004 equal to the previous peak rate in 1982. The age-adjusted percent increase between 1998 and 2004 was 35 percent. This overall increase was the net of diagnoses whose rates increased and diagnoses whose rates decreased. The largest contributor to the increase was "other digestive diseases"—those conditions that do not have separate chapters in this report. The largest individual disease contributions to the increase were made by gastroesophageal reflux disease (GERD), with an increase over this period of 376 per 100,000 population; viral hepatitis C, with 79 per 100,000; chronic constipation, with 62 per 100,000; intestinal infections, with 41 per 100,000; and pancreatitis, with 23 per 100,000. Except for pancreatitis, each of these diagnoses was more likely to be listed as a secondary discharge diagnosis than as the first-listed diagnosis.

The recent increase in overnight hospital stays with a diagnosis of digestive disease is surprising for two reasons. A few common conditions were known to have declined as reasons for overnight hospitalizations, notably peptic ulcer disease (due to decreased frequency) and gallstones (due to shift to same-day surgery). Of greater significance was the modest rate of increase of hospital discharges for all diseases (from 11,569 per 100,000 in 1998 to 13,104 per 100,000 in 2004, a 13.3 percent increase) relative to the larger increase for digestive diseases. In 1998, 25.3 percent of all hospital discharges had a diagnosis of digestive diseases; this increased to 30.1 percent in 2004. Thus, rates of hospitalizations with digestive disease diagnoses increased both absolutely and as a proportion of all hospitalizations.

In 2004, there were more than 236,000 deaths in the United States with a digestive disease as the underlying cause (Table 2), which represented 9.8 percent of all deaths. A disproportionately lower proportion of deaths from digestive diseases occurred among children (4.1 percent) and a higher proportion occurred among middle-aged adults (15.1 percent). There was no major variation in the distribution of deaths from digestive disease as a proportion of all deaths by race or sex. However, blacks had a 29 percent higher death rate than whites, and men had a 53 percent higher rate than women.

There were 2 million years of potential life lost (YPLL) prior to age 75 years due to digestive diseases, representing 8.5 years per death with digestive disease as an underlying cause. Digestive diseases were more frequently listed as underlying cause than as contributing cause, mainly due to the large effect of deaths from cancer, which was usually listed as underlying cause. There was a gradual decline in digestive disease mortality between 1979 and 2004, both as underlying (18.2 percent) and as underlying or other cause (20.3 percent) (Figure 2). There have been many contributions to this decline, but the greatest determinant was the decrease in digestive disease cancer mortality by 19.8 percent as underlying cause and 24.0 percent as underlying or other cause.

The 10 costliest prescription drugs from retail pharmacies for digestive diseases, according to the 2004 Verispan database (Appendix 2), are shown in Table 3. Dominating the prescription market at 50.7 percent of total number of prescriptions and 77.3 percent of total cost were five proton pump inhibitors, which were mainly prescribed for GERD. The other costliest medications were mesalamine (for inflammatory bowel disease), ranitidine (another anti-acid agent), tegaserod [for irritable bowel syndrome (IBS) and constipation], and ribavirin and peginterferon alfa_2a (for hepatitis C). A deficiency of the drug data is lack of information on nonprescription medications, complementary and alternative medications, infusions, and drugs administered in the hospital.

Summary data for individual digestive diseases are shown in Table 4, ordered by underlying cause of death and type of disease. Five diseases each caused more than 10,000 deaths. These were liver disease and four cancers, led by colorectal cancer. Two common causes of death were transmissible infectious diseases: gastrointestinal (GI) infections and viral hepatitis C. Chronic viral hepatitis is also believed to be a significant contributor to liver and bile duct cancers, which accounted for more than 11,000 deaths.

The YPLL prior to age 75 years is the addition of the number of years prior to age 75 at which deaths occur.

A death at age 55 years, for example, contributes 20 YPLL, while a death at age 75 years contributes none. Malignancies were responsible for 6 of the top 10 digestive diseases that contributed the most to YPLL (Table 4). Liver disease was the second leading cause of death (after colorectal cancer), but contributed the greatest number of YPLL. Also among the 10 leading causes of YPLL were hepatitis C and pancreatitis.

The distribution of burden of medical care for digestive diseases is notably different from mortality from digestive diseases. The six leading diseases with diagnosis noted at ambulatory care visits were GERD, chronic constipation, abdominal wall hernia, hemorrhoids, diverticular disease, and IBS. At least three of these (GERD, constipation, and IBS) are largely caused by disordered function of the GI tract, and diverticular disease also may be in part a consequence of dysfunction. The six most common digestive diseases diagnoses on hospital discharge records were GERD, diverticular disease, liver disease, constipation, gallstones, and peptic ulcer disease. The main difference between the records for hospital discharge diagnoses and ambulatory care diagnoses was the high numbers of diagnoses with liver disease and peptic ulcer disease, which can be life-threatening, and gallstones, which are a common reason for surgery. Because GERD and constipation should rarely lead to hospitalization, it must be assumed that when listed on discharge, they either contributed to the reason for hospitalization or were listed in thousands of discharges simply because they were so common.

[1] Everhart JE. Overview. In: Everhart JE, editor. *Digestive diseases in the United States: epidemiology and impact.* US Department of Health and Human Services, Public Health Service, National Institutes of Health, National Institute of Diabetes and Digestive and Kidney Diseases. Washington, DC: US Government Printing Office, 1994; NIH Publication No. 94-1447 pp. 1–53.

Table 1. All Digestive Diseases: Number and Age-Adjusted Rates of Ambulatory Care Visits and Hospital Discharges With First-Listed and All-Listed Diagnoses by Age, Race, and Sex in the United States, 2004

		AMBULATORY CARE VISITS				HOSPITAL DISCHARGES			
		First-Listed Diagnosis		All-Listed Diagnoses		First-Listed Diagnosis		All-Listed Diagnoses	
DEMOGRAPHIC CHARACTERISTICS		Number in Thousands	Rate per 100,000	Number in Thousands	Rate per 100,000	Number in Thousands	Rate per 100,000	Number in Thousands	Rate per 100,000
AGE (Years)	Under 15	10,951	18,010	15,170	24,948	331	544	2,321	3,817
	15–44	21,348	16,967	28,749	22,848	1,112	884	2,401	1,908
	45–64	21,430	30,314	32,434	45,880	1,362	1,926	3,489	4,935
	65+	18,342	50,483	28,437	78,268	1,779	4,897	5,313	14,622
RACE	White	59,506	24,317	85,798	34,953	3,526	1,412	10,242	4,108
	Black	8,733	24,076	13,339	37,784	531	1,655	1,702	5,142
SEX	Female	39,531	25,827	59,553	38,648	2,545	1,592	7,593	4,753
	Male	32,540	23,017	45,236	32,159	2,023	1,483	5,909	4,335
TOTAL		72,071	24,543	104,790	35,684	4,591	1,563	13,533	4,608

SOURCE: National Ambulatory Medical Care Survey (NAMCS) and National Hospital Ambulatory Medical Care Survey (NHAMCS) (3-year average, 2003–2005), and Healthcare Cost and Utilization Project Nationwide Inpatient Sample (HCUP NIS)

Figure 1. All Digestive Diseases: Age-Adjusted Rates of Ambulatory Care Visits and Hospital Discharges With All-Listed Diagnoses in the United States, 1979–2004

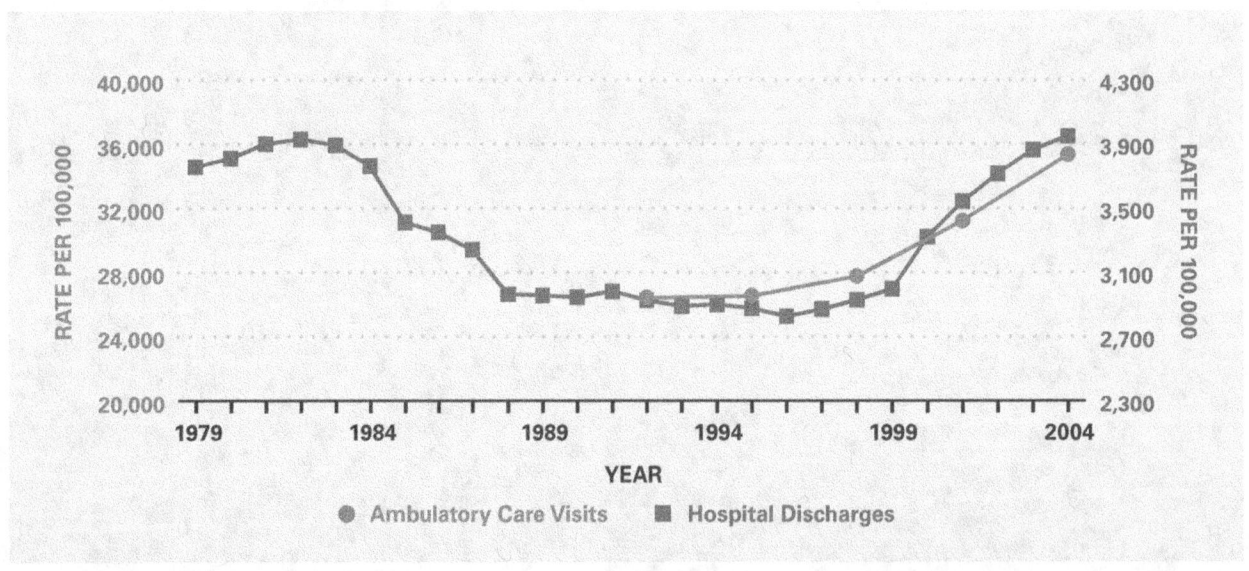

SOURCE: National Ambulatory Medical Care Survey (NAMCS) and National Hospital Ambulatory Medical Care Survey (NHAMCS) (averages 1992–1993, 1994–1996, 1997–1999, 2000–2002, 2003–2005), and National Hospital Discharge Survey (NHDS)

Table 2. All Digestive Diseases: Number and Age-Adjusted Rates of Deaths, Years of Potential Life Lost (to Age 75), and Digestive Disease as a Percentage of All Deaths by Age, Race, and Sex in the United States, 2004

DEMOGRAPHIC CHARACTERISTICS		UNDERLYING CAUSE				UNDERLYING OR OTHER CAUSE	
		Number of Deaths	Rate per 100,000	Years of Potential Life Lost in Thousands	Digestive Disease as a Percentage of All Deaths	Number of Deaths	Rate per 100,000
AGE (Years)	Under 15	1,612	2.7	118.2	4.1	2,908	4.8
	15–44	11,036	8.8	397.3	6.9	17,915	14.2
	45–64	66,806	94.5	1,263.8	15.1	92,862	131.4
	65+	156,706	431.3	228.2	8.9	252,709	695.5
RACE	White	200,834	77.0	1,579.4	9.8	313,055	119.7
	Black	27,812	99.5	340.2	9.7	42,514	152.7
SEX	Female	111,264	63.6	723.3	9.2	177,811	100.7
	Male	124,900	97.1	1,284.2	10.6	188,596	149.1
TOTAL		236,164	80.4	2,007.5	9.8	366,407	124.8

SOURCE: Vital Statistics of the United States

Figure 2. All Digestive Diseases: Age-Adjusted Rates of Death in the United States, 1979–2004

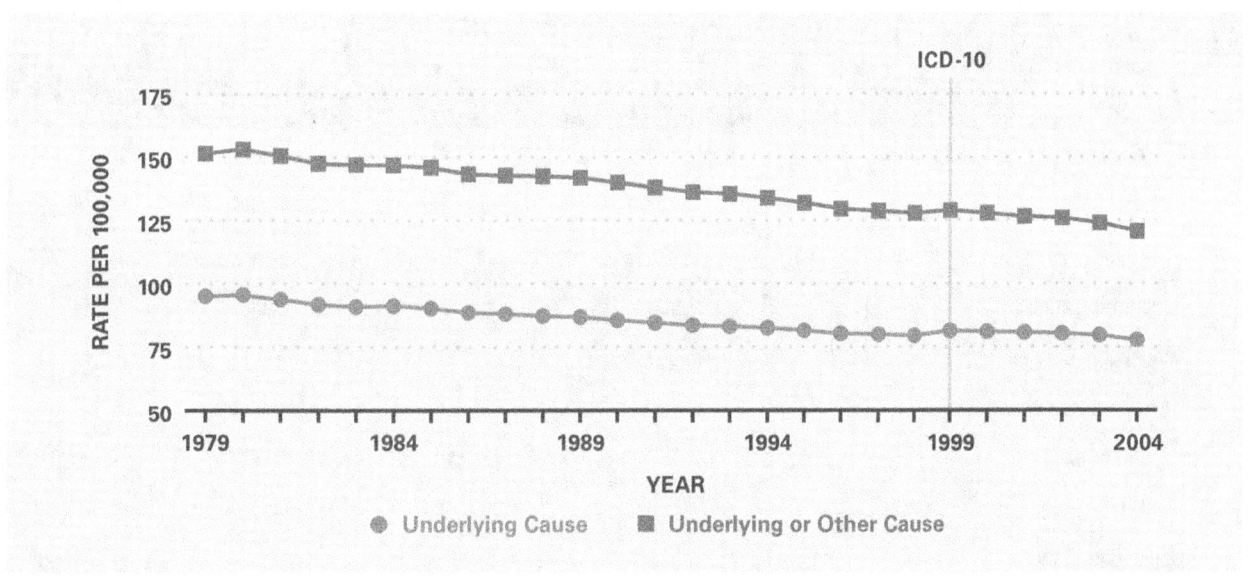

SOURCE: Vital Statistics of the United States

Table 3. All Digestive Diseases: Costliest Prescriptions

DRUG	Prescription (#)	Prescription	Retail Cost	Cost
Lansoprazole	20,989,993	15.5%	$3,104,963,208	25.2%
Esomeprazole	19,458,740	14.3	2,845,665,944	23.1
Pantoprazole	11,716,033	8.6	1,408,222,345	11.4
Rabeprazole	8,019,431	5.9	1,135,819,908	9.2
Omeprazole	8,582,644	6.3	1,038,622,087	8.4
Mesalamine	2,448,971	1.8	468,426,719	3.8
Ranitidine	13,171,338	9.7	319,418,374	2.6
Tegaserod	1,618,699	1.2	238,030,688	1.9
Ribavirin	221,035	0.2	229,351,616	1.9
Peginterferon alfa-2a	131,001	0.1	191,754,177	1.6
Other	49,378,593	36.4	1,351,443,116	11.0
TOTAL	135,736,478	100.0%	$12,331,718,182	100.0%

SOURCE: Verispan

Table 4. Burden of Selected Digestive Diseases in the United States, 2004

DIGESTIVE DISEASE	Deaths, Underlying Cause[a]	Years of Potential Life Lost to Age 75 Years[a]	Ambulatory Care Visits, All-Listed Diagnoses[b]	Hospital Discharges, All-Listed Diagnoses[c]
All Digestive Diseases	236,164	2,007,500	104,790,000	13,533,000
All Digestive Cancers	135,107	945,200	4,198,000	726,000
Colorectal Cancer	53,226	333,000	2,589,000	255,000
Pancreatic Cancer	31,800	206,800	415,000	68,000
Esophageal Cancer	13,667	113,800	372,000	44,000
Gastric Cancer	11,253	84,200	141,000	31,000
Primary Liver Cancer	6,323	72,400	63,000	33,000
Bile Duct Cancer	4,954	32,900	—	17,000
Gallbladder Cancer	1,939	10,900	—	6,000
Cancer of the Small Intestine	1,115	9,300	—	9,000
Liver Disease	36,090	559,100	2,398,000	759,000

Table 4. Burden of Selected Digestive Diseases in the United States, 2004 (continued)

DIGESTIVE DISEASE	Deaths, Underlying Cause[a]	Years of Potential Life Lost to Age 75 Years[a]	Ambulatory Care Visits, All-Listed Diagnoses[b]	Hospital Discharges, All-Listed Diagnoses[c]
All Viral Hepatitis	5,393	101,800	3,510,000	475,000
Hepatitis C	4,595	87,500	2,747,000	419,000
Hepatitis B	645	11,800	729,000	69,000
Hepatitis A	58	800	—	10,000
Gastrointestinal Infections	4,396	12,800	2,365,000	450,000
Peptic Ulcer Disease	3,692	19,700	1,473,000	489,000
Pancreatitis	3,480	42,800	881,000	454,000
Diverticular Disease	3,372	8,600	3,269,000	815,000
Abdominal Wall Hernia	1,172	6,900	4,787,000	372,000
Gastroesophageal Reflux Disease	1,150	6,000	18,342,000	3,189,000
Gallstones	1,092	4,400	1,836,000	622,000
All Inflammatory Bowel Disease	933	9,100	1,892,000	221,000
Crohn's Disease	622	7,000	1,176,000	141,000
Ulcerative Colitis	311	2,000	716,000	82,000
Appendicitis	453	5,000	782,000	325,000
All Functional Intestinal Disorders	423	2,500	11,648,000	1,241,000
Chronic Constipation	137	900	6,306,000	700,000
Irritable Bowel Syndrome	20	0	3,054,000	212,000
Hemorrhoids	14	200	3,275,000	306,000

SOURCE:[a] Vital Statistics of the United States
[b] National Ambulatory Medical Care Survey (NAMCS) and National Hospital Ambulatory Medical Care Survey (NHAMCS)
[c] Healthcare Cost and Utilization Project Nationwide Inpatient Sample (HCUP NIS)

CHAPTER 2
Gastrointestinal Infections
James E. Everhart, M.D., M.P.H.

Most GI infections are self-limited and do not come to medical attention, although they are both extremely common and disruptive of daily activities, including school and work. GI infections are caused by viral and bacterial pathogens, but the minority that are most severe and for which causative agents are found are typically bacterial. The ICD-9 and ICD-10 codes match well, except for nonspecified organisms. The most significant differences are that Intestinal Infections Due to Other Organisms (008) and Ill-Defined Intestinal Infections (009) in ICD-9 were replaced by Other Bacterial Intestinal Infections (A04), Other Bacterial Foodborne Intoxications (A05), and Viral and Other Specified Intestinal Infections (A08) in ICD-10. Here is a breakdown of the codes for GI infections:

	ICD-9	ICD-10
Cholera	001	A00
Typhoid and Paratyphoid	002	A01
Other Salmonella	003	A02
Shigellosis	004	A03
Other Food Poisoning	005	—
Other Bacterial Intestinal Infections	—	A04
Other Bacterial Foodborne Intoxications	—	A05
Amebiasis	006	A06
Other Protozoal Intestinal Diseases	007	A07
Intestinal Infections Due to Other Organisms	008	—
Viral and Other Specified Intestinal Infections	—	A08
Ill-Defined Intestinal Infections	009	—
Diarrhea and Gastroenteritis of Presumed Infectious Origin	—	A09
All GI Infections	001–009	A00–A09

As shown in Table 1, in 2004, more than half of ambulatory care visits for GI infections occurred in those under the age of 15 years. When first-listed, the rate in this age group (1,930 per 100,000 population), was at least 4 times that of any other age group. Age-adjusted rates were 45.7 percent higher among whites than blacks and 18.1 percent higher among females than males. Relative to the frequency of ambulatory care visits, hospitalizations were uncommon. In contrast to those in ambulatory care, persons over age 65 years had both the highest number and rate of hospitalizations, and blacks had rates similar to those of whites. GI infections were considerably more often a secondary diagnosis (272,000) than first-listed diagnosis (178,000). The rate of age-adjusted hospitalizations with a diagnosis of GI infections increased by 92.8 percent between 1979 (76.1 per 100,000) and 2004 (146.7 per 100,000) and by 43.3 percent between 1992 (102.4 per 100,000) and 2004 (Figure 1).

In 2004, there were 4,396 deaths with a GI infection listed as the underlying cause (Table 2). The large majority of these deaths occurred among persons age 65 years and older. The death rate among whites was 50 percent higher than that among blacks, and the rates were similar among females and males. Similar patterns were seen for GI infections as either underlying or contributing cause. Because the majority of deaths occurred in the elderly, the YPLL prior to age 75 years was small, less than 3 years per death. In recent years, there has been a remarkable increase in deaths from GI infections (Figure 2). Over the 20-year period between 1979 and 1999, the age-adjusted underlying cause mortality rate doubled from 0.21 per 100,000 to 0.42 per 100,000. But in the 5 years from 1999 to 2004, the rate more than tripled to 1.44 per 100,000. About two-thirds of the more recent increase is due to one bacterial cause, *Clostridium difficile*, which is coded under Other Bacterial Intestinal Infections as A04.7.

MEDICATIONS The costliest prescriptions filled at retail pharmacies for GI infections in 2004, according to the Verispan database (Appendix 2), are shown in Table 3. Most were antimicrobial agents, such as ciprofloxacin, or they affected GI motility, such as promethazine. An estimated 938,000 outpatient prescriptions were filled.

Table 1. Gastrointestinal Infections: Number and Age-Adjusted Rates of Ambulatory Care Visits and Hospital Discharges With First-Listed and All-Listed Diagnoses by Age, Race, and Sex in the United States, 2004

DEMOGRAPHIC CHARACTERISTICS		AMBULATORY CARE VISITS				HOSPITAL DISCHARGES			
		First-Listed Diagnosis		All-Listed Diagnoses		First-Listed Diagnosis		All-Listed Diagnoses	
		Number in Thousands	Rate per 100,000	Number in Thousands	Rate per 100,000	Number in Thousands	Rate per 100,000	Number in Thousands	Rate per 100,000
AGE (Years)	Under 15	1,174	1,930	1,222	2,010	47	77	83	137
	15–44	579	460	672	534	31	25	65	51
	45–64	266	377	311	440	34	47	86	122
	65+	109	301	159	439	66	183	215	593
RACE	White	1,800	785	1,994	867	140	57	359	144
	Black	225	529	253	595	16	46	48	151
SEX	Female	1,142	796	1,279	888	107	67	261	160
	Male	986	684	1,085	752	71	52	188	142
TOTAL		2,128	725	2,365	805	178	61	450	153

SOURCE: National Ambulatory Medical Care Survey (NAMCS) and National Hospital Ambulatory Medical Care Survey (NHAMCS) (3-year average, 2003–2005), and Healthcare Cost and Utilization Project Nationwide Inpatient Sample (HCUP NIS)

Figure 1. Gastrointestinal Infections: Age-Adjusted Rates of Ambulatory Care Visits and Hospital Discharges With All-Listed Diagnoses in the United States, 1979–2004

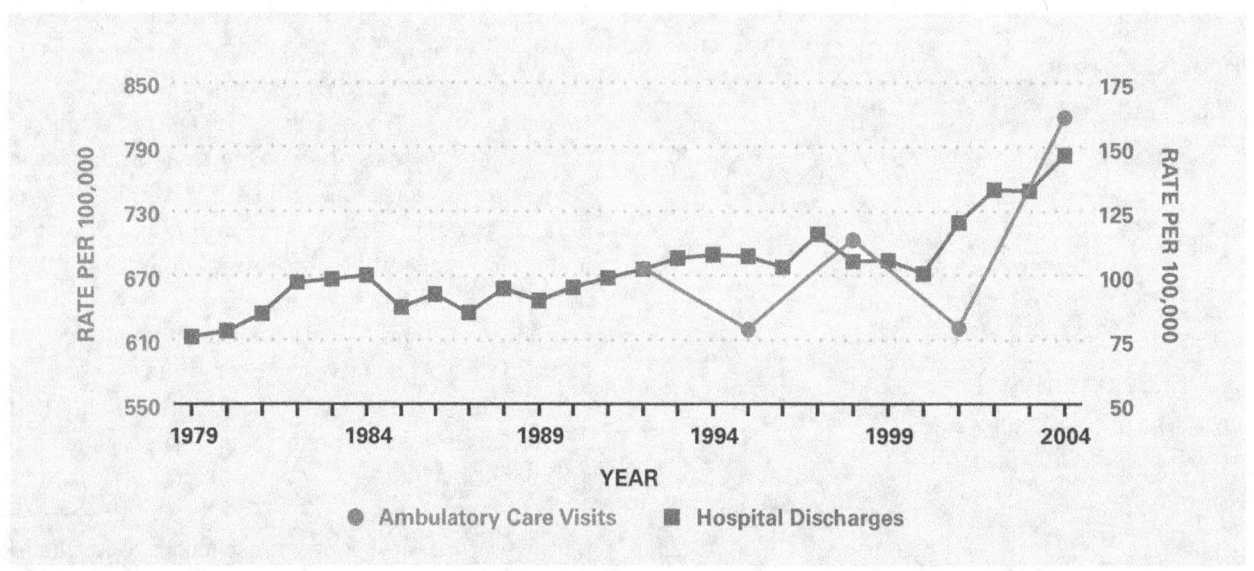

SOURCE: National Ambulatory Medical Care Survey (NAMCS) and National Hospital Ambulatory Medical Care Survey (NHAMCS) (averages 1992–1993, 1994–1996, 1997–1999, 2000–2002, 2003–2005), and National Hospital Discharge Survey (NHDS)

Table 2. Gastrointestinal Infections: Number and Age-Adjusted Rates of Deaths and Years of Potential Life Lost (to Age 75) by Age, Race, and Sex in the United States, 2004

DEMOGRAPHIC CHARACTERISTICS		UNDERLYING CAUSE			UNDERLYING OR OTHER CAUSE	
		Number of Deaths	Rate per 100,000	Years of Potential Life Lost in Thousands	Number of Deaths	Rate per 100,000
AGE (Years)	Under 15	32	0.1	2.3	40	0.1
	15–44	49	0.0	1.9	97	0.1
	45–64	353	0.5	6.0	577	0.8
	65+	3,962	10.9	2.6	6,345	17.5
RACE	White	4,104	1.5	10.7	6,552	2.5
	Black	241	1.0	1.6	422	1.6
SEX	Female	2,746	1.5	6.4	4,257	2.3
	Male	1,650	1.4	6.4	2,802	2.4
TOTAL		4,396	1.5	12.8	7,059	2.4

SOURCE: Vital Statistics of the United States

Figure 2. Gastrointestinal Infections: Age-Adjusted Rates of Death in the United States, 1979–2004

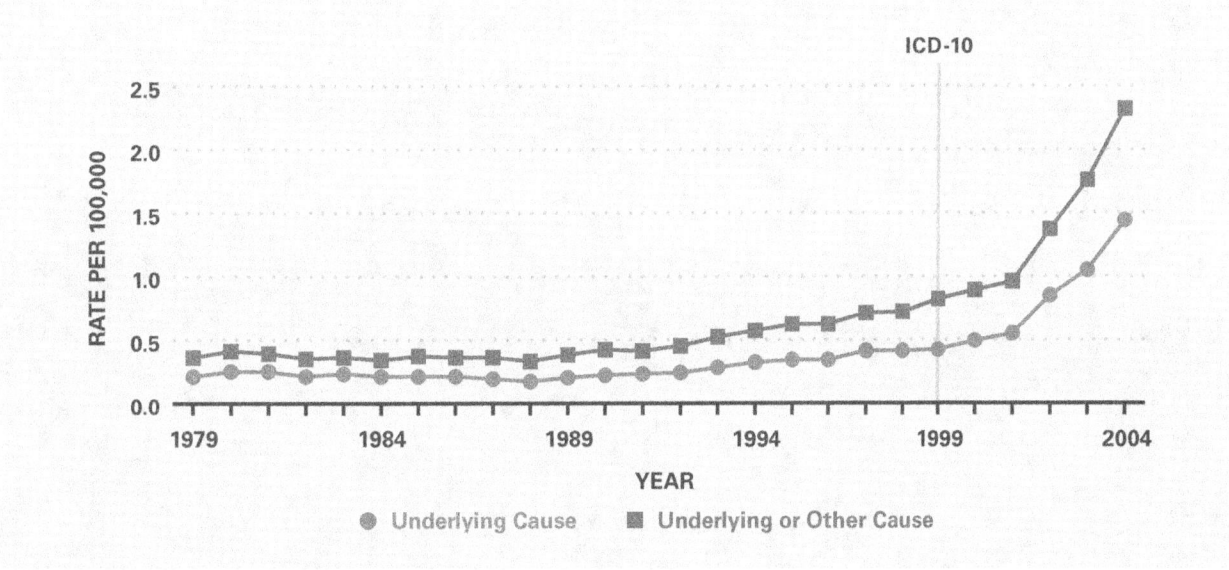

SOURCE: Vital Statistics of the United States

Table 3. Gastrointestinal Infections: Costliest Prescriptions

DRUG	Prescription (#)	Prescription	Retail Cost	Cost
Vancomycin	14,507	1.5%	$28,375,011	62.9%
Promethazine	346,794	37.0	5,985,173	13.3
Ciprofloxacin	126,523	13.4	5,132,893	11.4
Metronidazole	184,090	19.6	2,986,288	6.6
Loperamide	112,285	12.0	865,924	1.9
Diphenoxylate	122,042	13.0	832,096	1.8
Levofloxacin	7,325	0.8	483,046	1.1
Acidophilus/Bulgaricus	20,432	2.2	275,062	0.6
Ciprofloxacin-Betaine Combination	1,215	0.1	109,988	0.2
Prochlorperazine	2,927	0.3	26,326	0.1
Other	67	0.0	5,788	0.0
TOTAL	938,207	100.0%	$45,077,595	100.0%

SOURCE: Verispan

CHAPTER 3

Viral Hepatitis

James E. Everhart, M.D., M.P.H.

The primary forms of viral hepatitis in the United States are hepatitis A, B, and C (see ICD codes in Appendix 1). Hepatitis A is common and can be serious or even lethal. It does not have a chronic form. Hepatitis B can cause both acute and chronic disease, whereas acute hepatitis C is often asymptomatic, and its burden is predominantly due to chronic disease.

HEPATITIS A

Although the infection is common, hepatitis A is infrequently recognized in the ambulatory care or hospital setting. It was too infrequent to appear in the office-based sample of the National Ambulatory Medical Care Survey (Table 1). Hospitalization rates declined by about 75 percent between 1979 and 1993, and remained relatively stable through 2004. An effective vaccine to prevent infection was introduced in the 1990s, but it has not had a noticeable effect on reducing hospitalizations (Figure 1). Mortality from hepatitis A was rare, with fewer than 100 deaths per year (Table 2). Unlike recently stable rates of hospitalizations, the death rate from viral hepatitis A was halved between 1999 and 2004 (Figure 2).

HEPATITIS B

Viral hepatitis B is a more significant disease than hepatitis A. In the United States, infections were most commonly recognized between ages 15 and 44 years, and hospitalizations with the diagnosis occurred across the age range of adults (Table 3). Rates of both ambulatory care visits and hospitalizations with hepatitis B were higher among blacks than whites and among males than females. Hepatitis B was rarely the first-listed hospital diagnosis. There has been a vaccine available for hepatitis B since the 1980s, but the rates of both ambulatory care and hospitalizations have increased markedly since 1999 (Figure 3). This increase has been attributed to increased rates of immigration of chronic carriers of hepatitis B virus. Although not a common cause of death, viral hepatitis B resulted in about 10 times as many deaths as hepatitis A (Table 4). The majority of deaths with hepatitis B as

either underlying or contributing cause occurred in middle age, between age 45 and 64 years. As with other forms of infections, hepatitis B was more often listed as a contributing than as an underlying cause. Deaths from hepatitis B increased between 1979 and 1994, but mortality steadily declined thereafter, in spite of (or perhaps related to) the increased rates of medical care (Figure 4). As an underlying cause, rates in 2004 were similar to those in 1979, but as a contributing cause, rates were considerably higher in 2004 than they had been 25 years earlier. Age-adjusted mortality was higher among blacks than whites.

HEPATITIS C

The hepatitis C virus was discovered in 1989, and tests for it soon followed. Most prior cases of non-A, non-B hepatitis are believed to have been viral hepatitis C. In both the outpatient and inpatient setting, more than half the cases were in persons ages 45–64 years (Table 5). Rates were at least twice as high among blacks as whites and among males as females. Viral hepatitis C was rarely the first-listed diagnosis at hospital discharge, but was frequently listed as a secondary diagnosis. As a result, only 2.6 percent of hospital discharge diagnoses for hepatitis C listed it as the first-listed diagnosis. Where hepatitis C was not the first-listed diagnosis, the most common underlying (first-listed) causes were chronic liver disease and its sequelae (10.4 percent), mood disorders (4.5 percent), cellulitis (3.8 percent), complications of procedures (2.6 percent), pneumonia (2.5 percent), and HIV (2.4 percent). The majority of hospitalizations, however, appeared to be unrelated to hepatitis C, suggesting that the diagnoses may appear as a result of testing for hepatitis C, rather than as consequences of hepatitis C. Blacks and men had the highest age-adjusted rates.

Both outpatient and inpatient diagnoses have greatly increased since hepatitis C received its own ICD code in the early 1990s (Figure 5). The number of hospitalizations prior to 1992 was too small to provide estimates. Much of the increase can be attributed to increasing recognition of the disease. There was also the introduction of antiviral therapy that required frequent patient monitoring. It is not clear how much of the increase can be attributed to the consequences of disease burden due to longstanding infection.

In 2004, 85 percent of hepatitis-related deaths were from viral hepatitis C. Hepatitis C was listed as a contributing cause of death more often than as the underlying cause (Table 6). About two-thirds of deaths occurred between the ages of 45 and 64 years. Age-adjusted death rates among blacks were nearly twice those of whites, and males had more than double the death rate of females. Hepatitis C contributed a high number of YPLL before the age of 75 years (87,500), because of the large number of deaths and because few deaths are attributed to the disease after age 75. This number placed hepatitis C as the fifth leading digestive disease cause of YPLL, behind esophageal cancer and ahead of gastric cancer. In keeping with the growing identification and long-term consequences of the disease, mortality rates increased rapidly from 1990 to 2004 (Figure 6). (The few deaths recorded prior to 1990 were for non-A, non-B viral hepatitis.) Of note, the mortality rate for hepatitis C as underlying cause leveled off beginning in 2001 and as underlying or contributing cause in 2002.

ALL VIRAL HEPATITIS

The burden of all viral hepatitis primarily reflected that of hepatitis B in past years and, more recently, hepatitis C (Tables 7 and 8, Figures 7 and 8). For example, 97.5 percent of the YPLL prior to age 75 years due to viral hepatitis was a result of hepatitis B (11.6 percent) or hepatitis C (85.9 percent).

MEDICATIONS The costliest prescriptions filled at retail pharmacies for viral hepatitis in 2004, according to the Verispan database (Appendix 2), are shown in Table 9. An estimated 637,000 outpatient prescriptions were filled, but these were represented by few drugs, which were prescribed exclusively for hepatitis B (adefovir and lamivudine) or hepatitis C (ribavirin and peginterferon). When used to treat hepatitis C, ribavirin was nearly always used with interferon. For a full course of therapy, each of the medications in Table 9 would have required multiple prescriptions.

Table 1. Hepatitis A: Number and Age-Adjusted Rates of Ambulatory Care Visits and Hospital Discharges With First-Listed and All-Listed Diagnoses by Age, Race, and Sex in the United States, 2004

DEMOGRAPHIC CHARACTERISTICS		AMBULATORY CARE VISITS				HOSPITAL DISCHARGES			
		First-Listed Diagnosis		All-Listed Diagnoses		First-Listed Diagnosis		All-Listed Diagnoses	
		Number in Thousands	Rate per 100,000	Number in Thousands	Rate per 100,000	Number in Thousands	Rate per 100,000	Number in Thousands	Rate per 100,000
AGE (Years)	Under 15	—	—	—	—	0	1	0	1
	15–44	—	—	—	—	1	1	3	3
	45–64	—	—	—	—	0	1	4	5
	65+	—	—	—	—	0	1	2	6
RACE	White	—	—	—	—	2	1	7	3
	Black	—	—	—	—	0	0	2	4
SEX	Female	—	—	—	—	1	1	5	3
	Male	—	—	—	—	1	1	5	3
TOTAL		—	—	—	—	2	1	10	3

SOURCE: National Ambulatory Medical Care Survey (NAMCS) and National Hospital Ambulatory Medical Care Survey (NHAMCS) (3-year average, 2003–2005), and Healthcare Cost and Utilization Project Nationwide Inpatient Sample (HCUP NIS)

Figure 1. Hepatitis A: Age-Adjusted Rates of Ambulatory Care Visits and Hospital Discharges With All-Listed Diagnoses in the United States, 1979–2004 (Ambulatory Care Visit Data Unavailable)

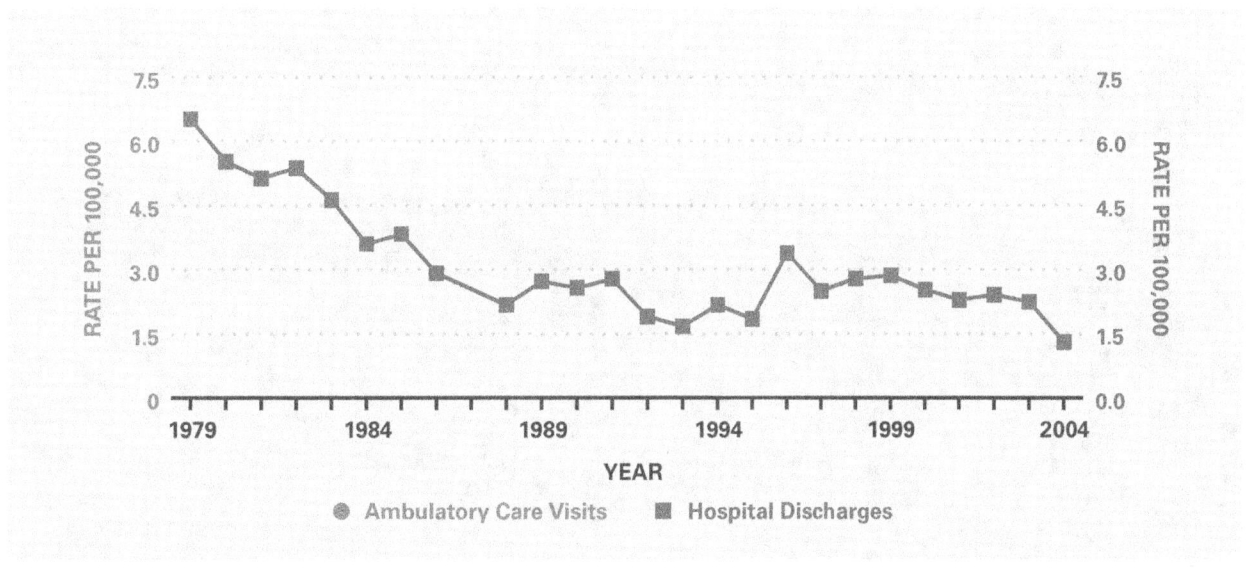

SOURCE: National Ambulatory Medical Care Survey (NAMCS) and National Hospital Ambulatory Medical Care Survey (NHAMCS) (averages 1992–1993, 1994–1996, 1997–1999, 2000–2002, 2003–2005), and National Hospital Discharge Survey (NHDS)

Table 2. Hepatitis A: Number and Age-Adjusted Rates of Deaths and Years of Potential Life Lost (to Age 75) by Age, Race, and Sex in the United States, 2004

DEMOGRAPHIC CHARACTERISTICS		UNDERLYING CAUSE			UNDERLYING OR OTHER CAUSE	
		Number of Deaths	Rate per 100,000	Years of Potential Life Lost in Thousands	Number of Deaths	Rate per 100,000
AGE (Years)	Under 15	—	—	—	—	—
	15–44	6	0.0	0.2	13	0.0
	45–64	27	0.0	0.6	61	0.1
	65+	25	0.1	0.0	55	0.2
RACE	White	48	0.0	0.7	101	0.0
	Black	7	0.0	0.1	20	0.1
SEX	Female	28	0.0	0.3	57	0.0
	Male	30	0.0	0.5	72	0.1
TOTAL		58	0.0	0.8	129	0.0

SOURCE: Vital Statistics of the United States

Figure 2. Hepatitis A: Age-Adjusted Rates of Death in the United States, 1979–2004

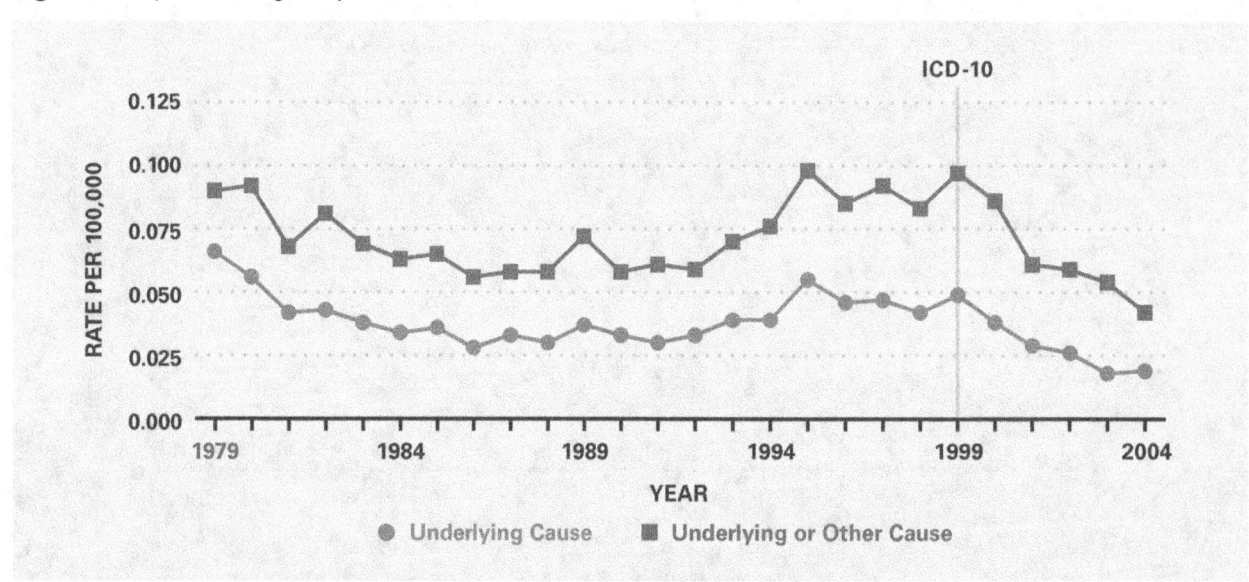

SOURCE: Vital Statistics of the United States

Table 3. Hepatitis B: Number and Age-Adjusted Rates of Ambulatory Care Visits and Hospital Discharges With First-Listed and All-Listed Diagnoses by Age, Race, and Sex in the United States, 2004

		AMBULATORY CARE VISITS				HOSPITAL DISCHARGES			
		First-Listed Diagnosis		All-Listed Diagnoses		First-Listed Diagnosis		All-Listed Diagnoses	
DEMOGRAPHIC CHARACTERISTICS		Number in Thousands	Rate per 100,000	Number in Thousands	Rate per 100,000	Number in Thousands	Rate per 100,000	Number in Thousands	Rate per 100,000
AGE (Years)	Under 15	—	—	—	—	—	—	—	—
	15–44	—	—	385	306	2	1	26	21
	45–64	—	—	277	392	1	2	33	47
	65+	—	—	—	—	0	1	9	26
RACE	White	—	—	242	98	2	1	40	16
	Black	—	—	183	510	1	3	19	55
SEX	Female	—	—	122	83	1	1	26	17
	Male	—	—	607	418	2	1	43	29
TOTAL		448	152	729	248	4	1	69	23

SOURCE: National Ambulatory Medical Care Survey (NAMCS) and National Hospital Ambulatory Medical Care Survey (NHAMCS) (3-year average, 2003–2005), and Healthcare Cost and Utilization Project Nationwide Inpatient Sample (HCUP NIS)

Figure 3. Hepatitis B: Age-Adjusted Rates of Ambulatory Care Visits and Hospital Discharges With All-Listed Diagnoses in the United States, 1979–2004

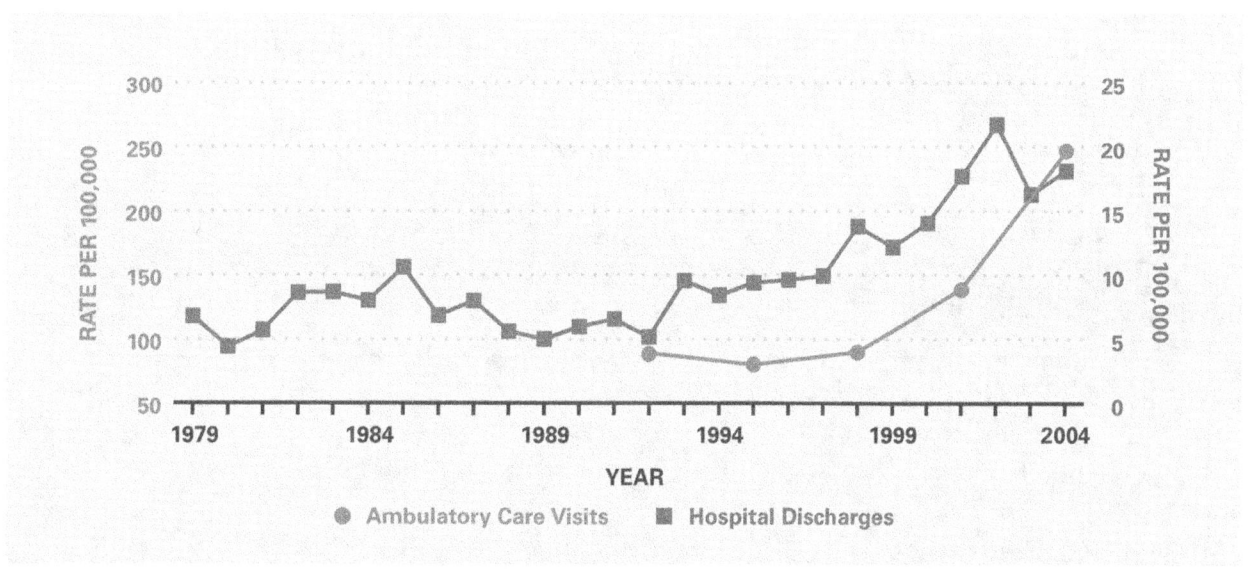

SOURCE: National Ambulatory Medical Care Survey (NAMCS) and National Hospital Ambulatory Medical Care Survey (NHAMCS) (averages 1992–1993, 1994–1996, 1997–1999, 2000–2002, 2003–2005), and National Hospital Discharge Survey (NHDS)

Table 4. Hepatitis B: Number and Age-Adjusted Rates of Deaths and Years of Potential Life Lost (to Age 75) by Age, Race, and Sex in the United States, 2004

DEMOGRAPHIC CHARACTERISTICS		UNDERLYING CAUSE			UNDERLYING OR OTHER CAUSE	
		Number of Deaths	Rate per 100,000	Years of Potential Life Lost in Thousands	Number of Deaths	Rate per 100,000
AGE (Years)	Under 15	—	—	—	1	0.0
	15–44	115	0.1	4.2	291	0.2
	45–64	346	0.5	7.1	962	1.4
	65+	184	0.5	0.5	441	1.2
RACE	White	424	0.2	7.6	984	0.4
	Black	124	0.4	2.5	390	1.2
SEX	Female	174	0.1	2.7	428	0.3
	Male	471	0.3	9.1	1,267	0.9
TOTAL		645	0.2	11.8	1,695	0.6

SOURCE: Vital Statistics of the United States

Figure 4. Hepatitis B: Age-Adjusted Rates of Death in the United States, 1979–2004

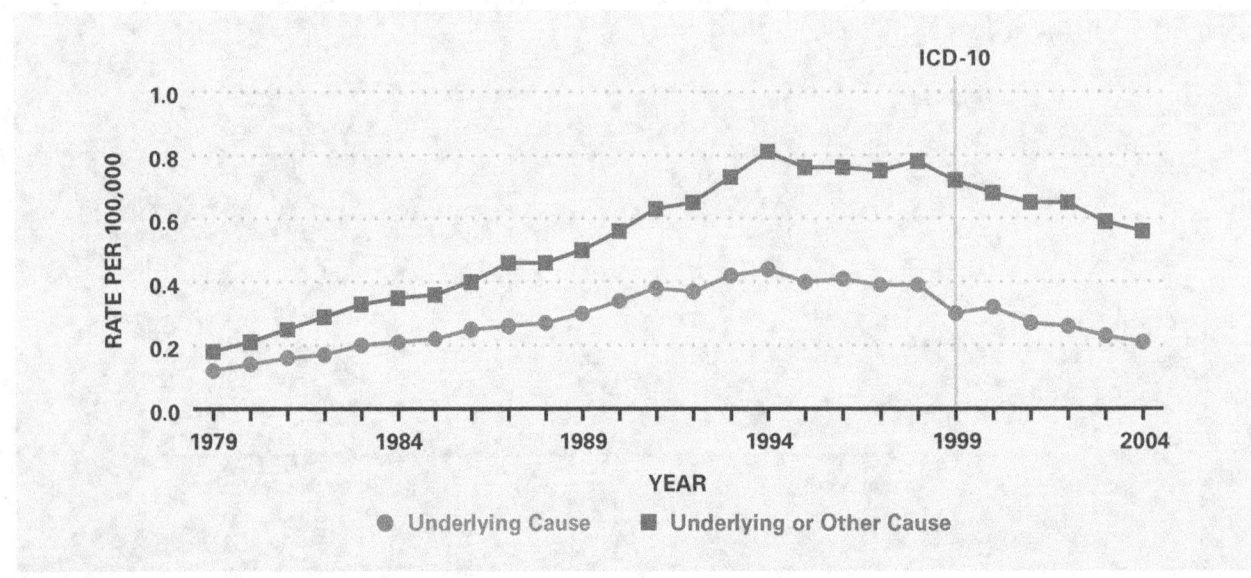

SOURCE: Vital Statistics of the United States

Table 5. Hepatitis C: Number and Age-Adjusted Rates of Ambulatory Care Visits and Hospital Discharges With First-Listed and All-Listed Diagnoses by Age, Race, and Sex in the United States, 2004

DEMOGRAPHIC CHARACTERISTICS		AMBULATORY CARE VISITS				HOSPITAL DISCHARGES			
		First-Listed Diagnosis		All-Listed Diagnoses		First-Listed Diagnosis		All-Listed Diagnoses	
		Number in Thousands	Rate per 100,000	Number in Thousands	Rate per 100,000	Number in Thousands	Rate per 100,000	Number in Thousands	Rate per 100,000
AGE (Years)	Under 15	—	—	—	—	—	—	0	0
	15–44	382	304	791	628	2	2	127	101
	45–64	918	1,298	1,603	2,268	7	10	248	351
	65+	—	—	353	970	1	4	43	118
RACE	White	1,110	451	1,828	742	9	3	298	120
	Black	235	662	739	2,122	2	5	99	286
SEX	Female	514	331	925	604	4	3	161	105
	Male	974	677	1,823	1,261	7	4	258	176
TOTAL		1,487	506	2,747	936	11	4	419	143

SOURCE: National Ambulatory Medical Care Survey (NAMCS) and National Hospital Ambulatory Medical Care Survey (NHAMCS) (3-year average, 2003–2005), and Healthcare Cost and Utilization Project Nationwide Inpatient Sample (HCUP NIS)

Figure 5. Hepatitis C: Age-Adjusted Rates of Ambulatory Care Visits and Hospital Discharges With All-Listed Diagnoses in the United States, 1979–2004

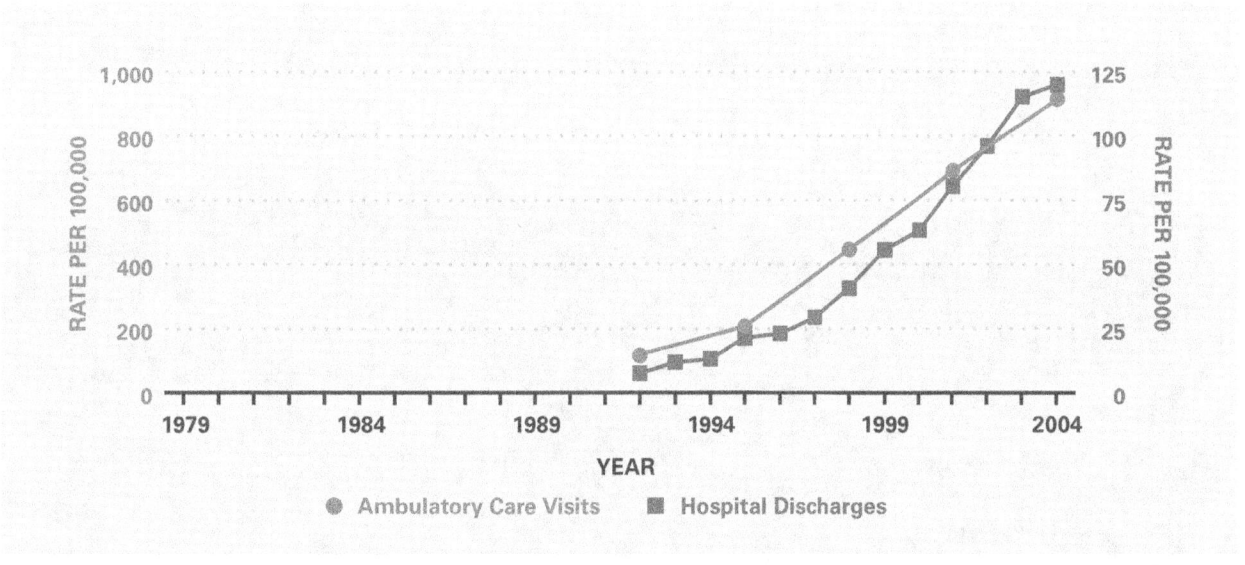

SOURCE: National Ambulatory Medical Care Survey (NAMCS) and National Hospital Ambulatory Medical Care Survey (NHAMCS) (averages 1992–1993, 1994–1996, 1997–1999, 2000–2002, 2003–2005), and National Hospital Discharge Survey (NHDS)

Table 6. Hepatitis C: Number and Age-Adjusted Rates of Deaths and Years of Potential Life Lost (to Age 75) by Age, Race, and Sex in the United States, 2004

DEMOGRAPHIC CHARACTERISTICS		UNDERLYING CAUSE			UNDERLYING OR OTHER CAUSE	
		Number of Deaths	Rate per 100,000	Years of Potential Life Lost in Thousands	Number of Deaths	Rate per 100,000
AGE (Years)	Under 15	2	0.0	0.1	3	0.0
	15–44	547	0.4	18.6	1,445	1.1
	45–64	3,062	4.3	66.1	7,590	10.7
	65+	984	2.7	2.7	2,253	6.2
RACE	White	3,712	1.4	71.0	8,771	3.4
	Black	718	2.2	14.2	2,111	6.4
SEX	Female	1,625	1.0	26.8	3,448	2.2
	Male	2,970	2.0	60.8	7,844	5.3
TOTAL		4,595	1.6	87.5	11,292	3.8

SOURCE: Vital Statistics of the United States

Figure 6. Hepatitis C: Age-Adjusted Rates of Death in the United States, 1979–2004

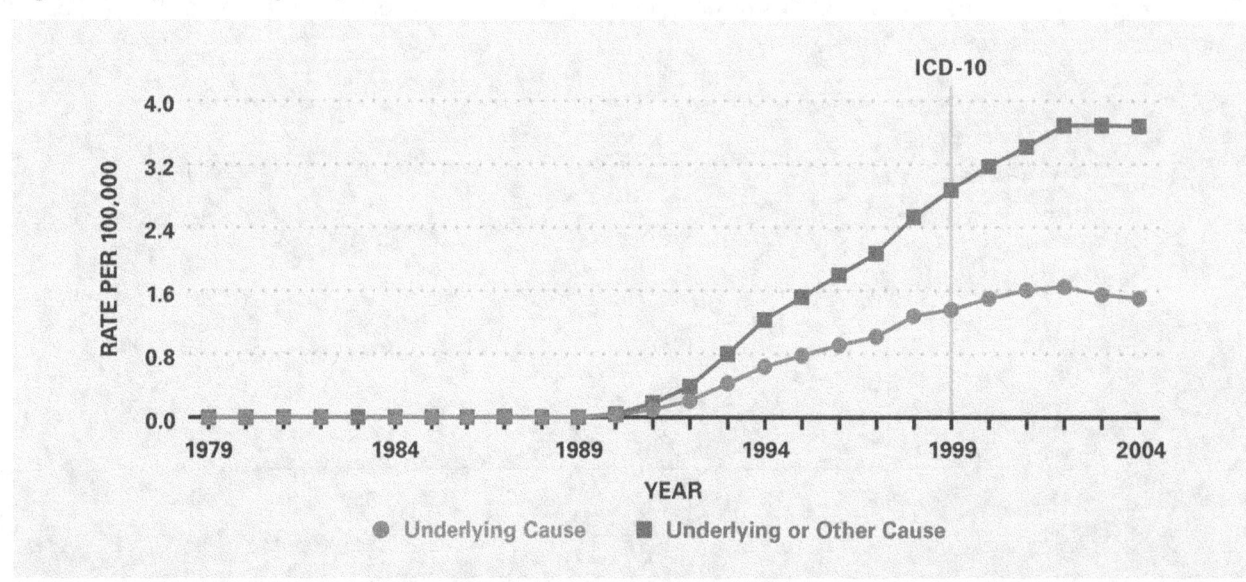

SOURCE: Vital Statistics of the United States

Table 7. All Viral Hepatitis: Number and Age-Adjusted Rates of Ambulatory Care Visits and Hospital Discharges With First-Listed and All-Listed Diagnoses by Age, Race, and Sex in the United States, 2004

DEMOGRAPHIC CHARACTERISTICS		AMBULATORY CARE VISITS				HOSPITAL DISCHARGES			
		First-Listed Diagnosis		All-Listed Diagnoses		First-Listed Diagnosis		All-Listed Diagnoses	
		Number in Thousands	Rate per 100,000	Number in Thousands	Rate per 100,000	Number in Thousands	Rate per 100,000	Number in Thousands	Rate per 100,000
AGE (Years)	Under 15	—	—	—	—	1	1	1	2
	15–44	627	499	1,174	933	6	5	150	119
	45–64	1,118	1,582	1,914	2,708	10	14	271	383
	65+	—	—	399	1,099	2	6	53	147
RACE	White	1,260	509	2,101	852	14	6	330	133
	Black	315	869	919	2,625	3	9	113	326
SEX	Female	620	404	1,071	703	8	5	185	121
	Male	1,356	936	2,439	1,685	11	7	290	198
TOTAL		1,977	673	3,510	1,195	19	6	475	162

SOURCE: National Ambulatory Medical Care Survey (NAMCS) and National Hospital Ambulatory Medical Care Survey (NHAMCS) (3-year average, 2003–2005), and Healthcare Cost and Utilization Project Nationwide Inpatient Sample (HCUP NIS)

Figure 7. All Viral Hepatitis: Age-Adjusted Rates of Ambulatory Care Visits and Hospital Discharges With All-Listed Diagnoses in the United States, 1979–2004

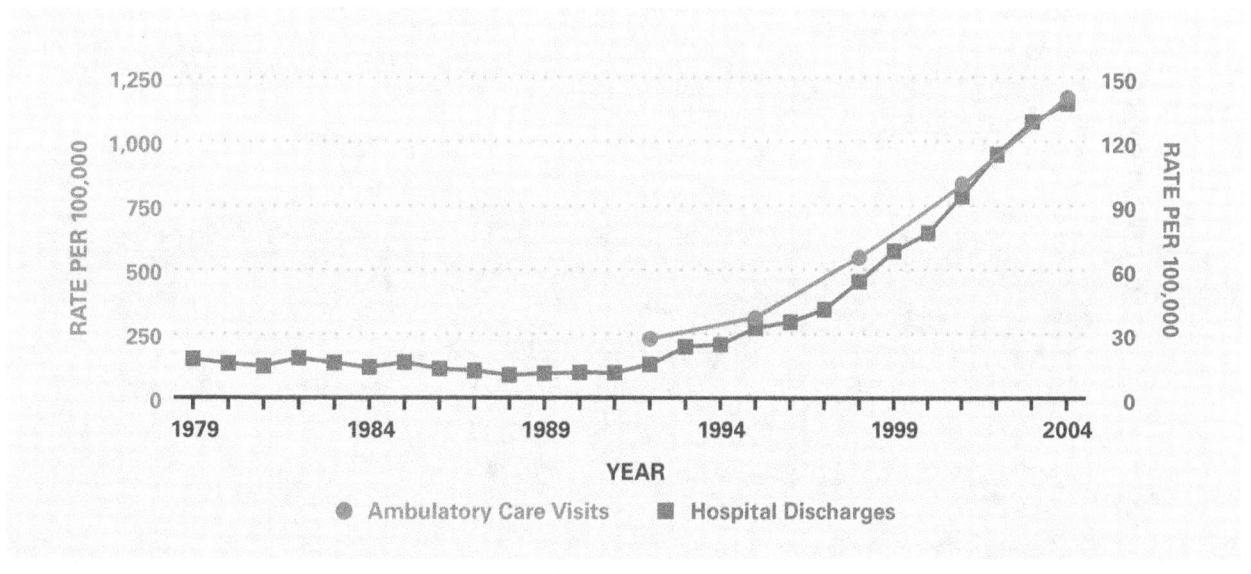

SOURCE: National Ambulatory Medical Care Survey (NAMCS) and National Hospital Ambulatory Medical Care Survey (NHAMCS) (averages 1992–1993, 1994–1996, 1997–1999, 2000–2002, 2003–2005), and National Hospital Discharge Survey (NHDS)

Table 8. All Viral Hepatitis: Number and Age-Adjusted Rates of Deaths and Years of Potential Life Lost (to Age 75) by Age, Race, and Sex in the United States, 2004

DEMOGRAPHIC CHARACTERISTICS		UNDERLYING CAUSE			UNDERLYING OR OTHER CAUSE	
		Number of Deaths	Rate per 100,000	Years of Potential Life Lost in Thousands	Number of Deaths	Rate per 100,000
AGE (Years)	Under 15	3	0.0	0.2	9	0.0
	15–44	684	0.5	23.7	1,674	1.3
	45–64	3,477	4.9	74.7	8,249	11.7
	65+	1,229	3.4	3.2	2,723	7.5
RACE	White	4,254	1.7	80.4	9,538	3.7
	Black	866	2.6	17.1	2,401	7.3
SEX	Female	1,872	1.2	30.5	3,850	2.4
	Male	3,521	2.4	71.3	8,806	6.0
TOTAL		5,393	1.8	101.8	12,656	4.3

SOURCE: Vital Statistics of the United States

Figure 8. All Viral Hepatitis: Age-Adjusted Rates of Death in the United States, 1979–2004

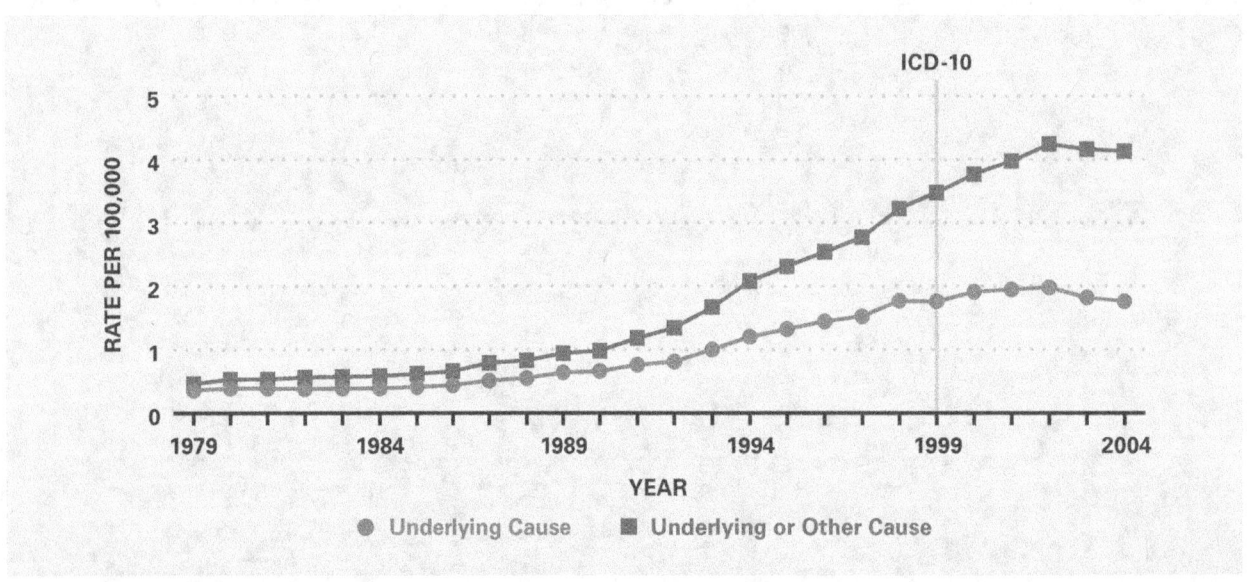

SOURCE: Vital Statistics of the United States

Table 9. All Viral Hepatitis: Costliest Prescriptions

DRUG	Prescription (#)	Prescription	Retail Cost	Cost
Ribavirin	221,035	34.7%	$229,351,616	40.0%
Peginterferon alfa-2a	131,001	20.5	191,754,177	33.5
Peginterferon alfa-2b	64,398	10.1	84,943,979	14.8
Adefovir	86,784	13.6	43,120,493	7.5
Lamivudine	134,657	21.1	23,580,159	4.2
TOTAL	637,875	100.0%	$572,750,424	100.0%

SOURCE: Verispan

CHAPTER 4

Digestive Cancers

James E. Everhart, M.D., M.P.H.

The Surveillance, Epidemiology, and End Results (SEER) program provides considerable information on cancer burden not available for other digestive diseases. SEER statistics used in this report are number of cases and incidence in 2004, and the time trends for incidence and 5-year survival following diagnosis between 1979 and 2004. The codes used by ICD-9, ICD-10, and SEER are listed in Appendix 1.

ALL DIGESTIVE SYSTEM CANCERS

In 2004, approximately 233,000 persons were diagnosed with digestive system cancers (Table 1), which represented 18 percent of all cancers and was second only to genital system cancers for the most commonly affected organ system. Two-thirds of digestive system cancers occurred among persons age 65 years and older. The median age of diagnosis was 70 years, compared with 67 years for all cancers (http://seer.cancer.gov/csr/1975_2005/results_merged/topic_med_age.pdf). Age-adjusted rates were highest among non-Hispanic blacks and lowest among American Indians. Males had slightly higher rates than females. Age-adjusted incidence declined by 13.2 percent between 1979 and 2004, with the entire decline coming after 1986 (Figure 1). Survival for all cancers and for individual cancers was calculated as absolute survival. Other reports may calculate survival relative to the general population with the same age and sex distribution, which would result in higher apparent survival. The same trends, however, would be seen for either approach. Five-year survival increased an absolute 6 percent to 34.6 percent; thus, for every 100 persons diagnosed with a digestive system cancer in 1999, 6 more survived at least 5 years longer than did those diagnosed 20 years earlier.

There were approximately 3.5 million ambulatory care visits for first-listed digestive system cancer in 2004 and 4.2 million all-listed visits. The elderly, whites, and males had the highest rates of ambulatory care visits (Table 2). Among all hospital discharges with digestive system cancers, about half were first-listed. The main demographic difference between ambulatory care diagnoses and hospital diagnoses was that blacks had a higher age-adjusted rate of hospital diagnoses. Rates of ambulatory care visits for digestive system cancers did not change appreciably over the period 1992–2004, but hospitalizations rates declined by 13.6 percent over that period (Figure 2).

In 2004, there were approximately 135,000 deaths due to digestive system cancers (Table 3), which represented 24 percent of all cancers and were second only to respiratory system cancers as cause of death due to cancer. As underlying cause, digestive system cancers constituted 57.2 percent of all digestive disease deaths. Death rates among persons 65 years and older were 5 times that of those aged 45–64 years. Age-adjusted death rates were higher among blacks and men. There were 945,000 YPLL due to digestive system cancer, the large majority occurring among males. Death rates from digestive system cancer declined steadily between 1979 and 2004 by an overall 19.8 percent (Figure 3).

MEDICATIONS The costliest prescriptions filled at retail pharmacies for digestive system malignancies in 2004, according to the Verispan database (Appendix 2), are shown in Table 4. An estimated 879,000 outpatient prescriptions were filled. The costliest agents were either anti-neoplastic agents, such as capecitabine, or nonspecific pain and anti-nausea medications, such as fentanyl. Because the prescriptions were filled at retail pharmacies and do not capture all the settings where anti-cancer treatment is prescribed, this table both underestimates the number of prescriptions and likely misses many of the drugs used to treat digestive system malignancies. Medications are not shown for the individual malignancies in the following chapters.

Table 1. All Digestive Cancers: Number of Cases and Incidence Rates by Age, Race/Ethnicity, and Sex, 2004

DEMOGRAPHIC CHARACTERISTICS		Number of Cases	INCIDENCE PER 100,000	
			Unadjusted	Age-Adjusted
AGE (Years)	Under 15	293	0.5	—
	15–44	10,927	9.1	—
	45–64	78,215	111.6	—
	65+	154,886	452.8	—
RACE/ETHNICITY	Non-Hispanic White	191,668	99.6	83.5
	Non-Hispanic Black	26,748	78.3	109.0
	Hispanic	15,921	39.3	81.8
	Asian/Pacific Islander	8,914	72.4	84.4
	American Indian/Alaska Native	1,009	54.5	75.0
SEX	Female	109,058	74.7	70.0
	Male	123,967	88.7	105.1
TOTAL		233,239	81.6	—

SOURCE: Surveillance, Epidemiology, and End Results (SEER) Program

Figure 1. All Digestive Cancers: Age-Adjusted Incidence Rates and 5-Year Survival Rates, 1979–2004

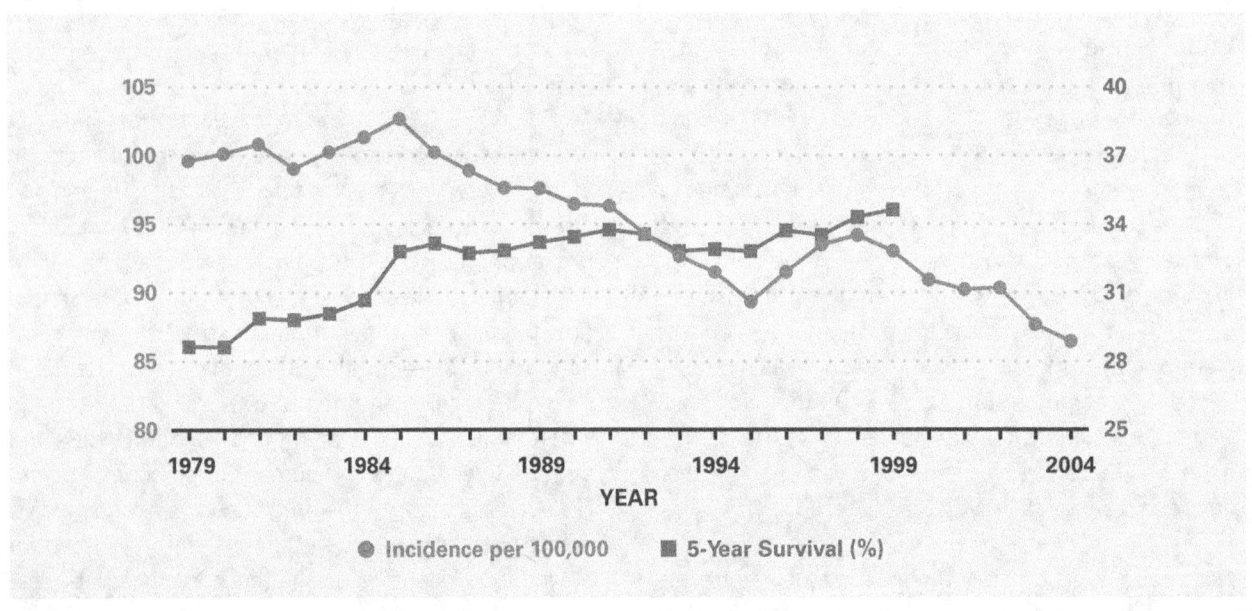

SOURCE: Surveillance, Epidemiology, and End Results (SEER) Program

Table 2. All Digestive Cancers: Number and Age-Adjusted Rates of Ambulatory Care Visits and Hospital Discharges With First-Listed and All-Listed Diagnoses by Age, Race, and Sex in the United States, 2004

DEMOGRAPHIC CHARACTERISTICS		AMBULATORY CARE VISITS				HOSPITAL DISCHARGES			
		First-Listed Diagnosis		All-Listed Diagnoses		First-Listed Diagnosis		All-Listed Diagnoses	
		Number in Thousands	Rate per 100,000	Number in Thousands	Rate per 100,000	Number in Thousands	Rate per 100,000	Number in Thousands	Rate per 100,000
AGE (Years)	Under 15	—	—	—	—	1	1	5	7
	15–44	110	87	145	115	19	15	47	37
	45–64	1,293	1,829	1,537	2,174	115	163	257	364
	65+	2,034	5,600	2,472	6,805	200	550	418	1,149
RACE	White	3,149	1,235	3,771	1,479	263	102	572	222
	Black	240	802	313	1,040	40	141	89	307
SEX	Female	1,740	1,081	2,218	1,375	167	100	374	226
	Male	1,741	1,309	1,980	1,485	168	128	351	267
TOTAL		3,481	1,185	4,198	1,429	335	114	726	247

SOURCE: National Ambulatory Medical Care Survey (NAMCS) and National Hospital Ambulatory Medical Care Survey (NHAMCS) (3-year average, 2003–2005), and Healthcare Cost and Utilization Project Nationwide Inpatient Sample (HCUP NIS)

Figure 2. All Digestive Cancers: Age-Adjusted Rates of Ambulatory Care Visits and Hospital Discharges With All-Listed Diagnoses in the United States, 1979–2004

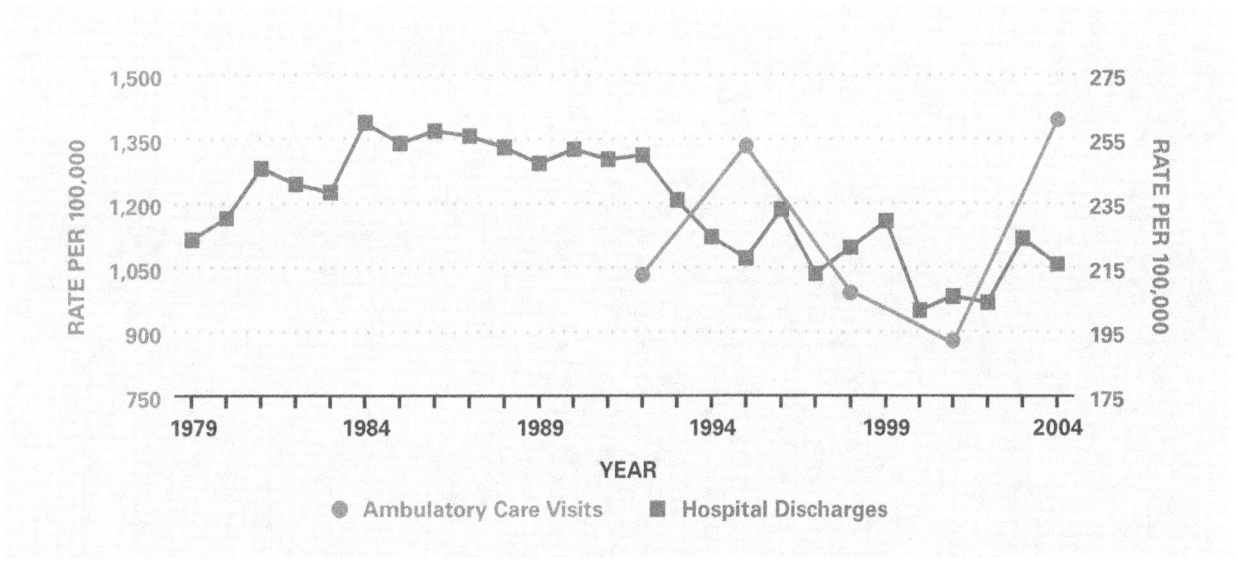

SOURCE: National Ambulatory Medical Care Survey (NAMCS) and National Hospital Ambulatory Medical Care Survey (NHAMCS) (averages 1992–1993, 1994–1996, 1997–1999, 2000–2002, 2003–2005), and National Hospital Discharge Survey (NHDS)

Table 3. All Digestive Cancers: Number and Age-Adjusted Rates of Deaths and Years of Potential Life Lost (to Age 75) by Age, Race, and Sex in the United States, 2004

DEMOGRAPHIC CHARACTERISTICS		UNDERLYING CAUSE			UNDERLYING OR OTHER CAUSE	
		Number of Deaths	Rate per 100,000	Years of Potential Life Lost in Thousands	Number of Deaths	Rate per 100,000
AGE (Years)	Under 15	43	0.1	3.0	57	0.1
	15–44	3,972	3.2	142.7	4,549	3.6
	45–64	35,968	50.9	648.1	41,599	58.8
	65+	95,123	261.8	151.5	114,984	316.5
RACE	White	113,468	43.5	737.8	136,231	52.2
	Black	16,907	62.2	161.7	19,587	72.3
SEX	Female	61,515	35.4	346.5	74,315	42.7
	Male	73,592	57.9	598.7	86,876	68.8
TOTAL		135,107	46.0	945.2	161,191	54.9

SOURCE: Vital Statistics of the United States

Figure 3. All Digestive Cancers: Age-Adjusted Rates of Death in the United States, 1979–2004

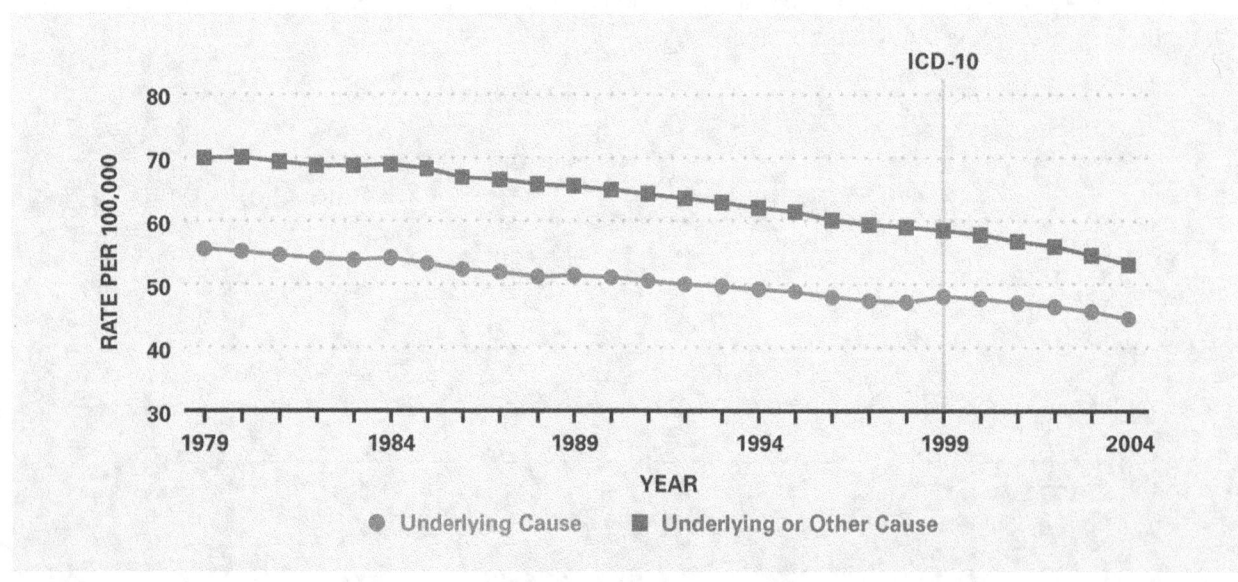

SOURCE: Vital Statistics of the United States

Table 4. All Digestive Cancers: Costliest Prescriptions

DRUG	Prescription (#)	Prescription	Retail Cost	Cost
Capecitabine	77,376	8.8%	$76,943,103	53.6%
Fentanyl	80,768	9.2	21,519,990	15.0
Oxycodone	92,577	10.5	20,027,456	14.0
Hydromorphone	371,312	42.2	16,110,590	11.2
Oxycodone/Acetaminophen	215,506	24.5	4,516,077	3.1
Morphine	17,890	2.0	3,690,323	2.6
Gemcitabine	379	0.0	361,858	0.3
Hydrocodone/Acetaminophen	4,285	0.5	249,901	0.2
Bevacizumab	18	0.0	45,962	0.0
Cetuximab	15	0.0	27,876	0.0
Other	18,557	2.0	14,683	0.0
TOTAL	878,683	100.0%	$143,507,819	100.0%

SOURCE: Verispan

CHAPTER 5

Cancer of the Esophagus

James E. Everhart, M.D., M.P.H.

The two forms of esophageal cancer are squamous cell carcinoma, which occurs in the upper two-thirds of the esophagus, and adenocarcinoma, which occurs in the lower part of the esophagus. Because the epidemiology of the two cancers is quite different, the SEER results are presented separately. Other national data sources do not differentiate as well, and those data therefore are combined.

In 2004, the majority (67 percent) of new cases of esophageal squamous cell cancer occurred among persons 65 years and older (Table 1) and occurred most often among non-Hispanic blacks and males (61 percent). The incidence declined over 25 years to 2004, when it was about half the rate of 1979 (Figure 1). Five-year survival remained poor, but improved from about 3 percent to 12 percent over that period.

Esophageal adenocarcinoma had a younger age distribution than most other digestive system cancers, but the majority of cases (63 percent) still occurred at age 65 years and older (Table 2). Non-Hispanic whites and males had by far the highest risk. These race and sex differences were greater than for any other common digestive tract cancer. During the 25 years of observation, the incidence of esophageal adenocarcinoma increased more rapidly than any other common malignancy, rising approximately fivefold between 1979 and 2004 (Figure 2). Five-year survival remained poor, but had increased from less than 5 percent to more than 15 percent.

Combining the two esophageal cancers (Table 3 and Figure 3) obscures their dynamic differences. For example, incidence of all esophageal cancer increased modestly over the period, but in 1979, adenocarcinoma was about one-eighth as frequent as squamous cell carcinoma, whereas by 2004, adenocarcinoma had the higher incidence. These combined data can, however, be useful for comparison with other national data. In 2004, there were an estimated 372,000 ambulatory care visits and 44,000 hospital diagnoses for esophageal cancer; rates of ambulatory care visits were moderately higher among persons age 65 years and older (Table 4). There were only sufficient numbers of ambulatory care visits for whites and males to show in the table. Hospitalizations occurred predominantly among persons age 65 years and older. During the 25 years of reporting, the rates of hospitalization remained relatively stable, in keeping with the overall incidence figures (Figure 4). Ambulatory care visits were too uncommon to discern a trend.

Esophageal cancer was a frequent cause of cancer death, ranking third in 2004 among digestive system cancers (after colorectal and pancreatic cancer) and was responsible for more than 13,000 deaths (Table 5) and 113,000 YPLL prior to age 75 years. Cancers of the gastroesophageal junction and cardia accounted for 4.6 percent of these deaths (see Chapter 6, Cancer of the Stomach). In keeping with the SEER data, death rates were highest among persons age 65 years and older, blacks (modestly more than whites), and males. Death rates increased between 1979 and 2004, but not during the last 6 years of that period.

Table 1. Esophageal Squamous Cell Cancer: Number of Cases and Incidence Rates by Age, Race/Ethnicity, and Sex, 2004

DEMOGRAPHIC CHARACTERISTICS		Number of Cases	INCIDENCE PER 100,000	
			Unadjusted	Age-Adjusted
AGE (Years)	Under 15	—	—	—
	15–44	94	0.1	—
	45–64	1,655	2.4	—
	65+	3,093	9.0	—
RACE/ETHNICITY	Non-Hispanic White	3,183	1.7	1.4
	Non-Hispanic Black	1,108	3.2	4.4
	Hispanic	263	0.7	1.4
	Asian/Pacific Islander	210	1.7	2.0
	American Indian/Alaska Native	—	—	—
SEX	Female	1,771	1.2	1.2
	Male	2,828	2.0	2.4
TOTAL		4,612	1.6	—

SOURCE: Surveillance, Epidemiology, and End Results (SEER) Program

Figure 1. Esophageal Squamous Cell Cancer: Age-Adjusted Incidence Rates and 5-Year Survival Rates, 1979–2004

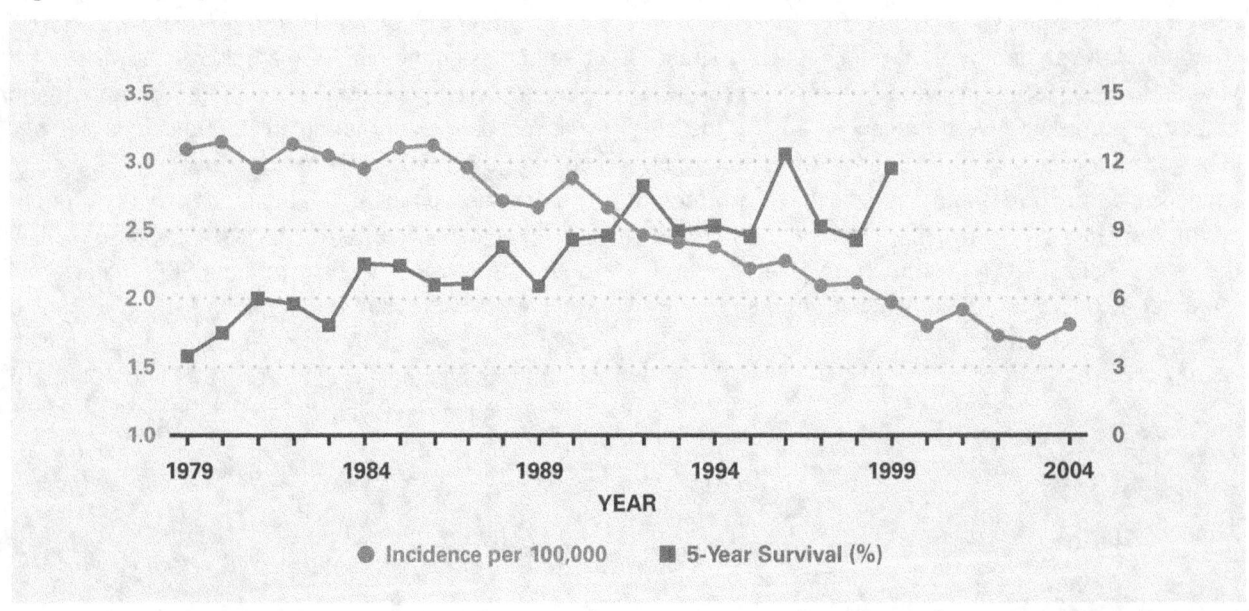

SOURCE: Surveillance, Epidemiology, and End Results (SEER) Program

Table 2. Esophageal Adenocarcinoma: Number of Cases and Incidence Rates by Age, Race/Ethnicity, and Sex, 2004

DEMOGRAPHIC CHARACTERISTICS		Number of Cases	INCIDENCE PER 100,000	
			Unadjusted	Age-Adjusted
AGE (Years)	Under 15	—	—	—
	15–44	198	0.2	—
	45–64	2,420	3.5	—
	65+	3,996	11.7	—
RACE/ETHNICITY	Non-Hispanic White	6,553	3.4	2.9
	Non-Hispanic Black	143	0.4	0.5
	Hispanic	268	0.7	1.4
	Asian/Pacific Islander	54	0.4	0.5
	American Indian/Alaska Native	—	—	—
SEX	Female	942	0.6	0.6
	Male	5,318	3.8	4.5
TOTAL		6,309	2.2	—

SOURCE: Surveillance, Epidemiology, and End Results (SEER) Program

Figure 2. Esophageal Adenocarcinoma: Age-Adjusted Incidence Rates and 5-Year Survival Rates, 1979–2004

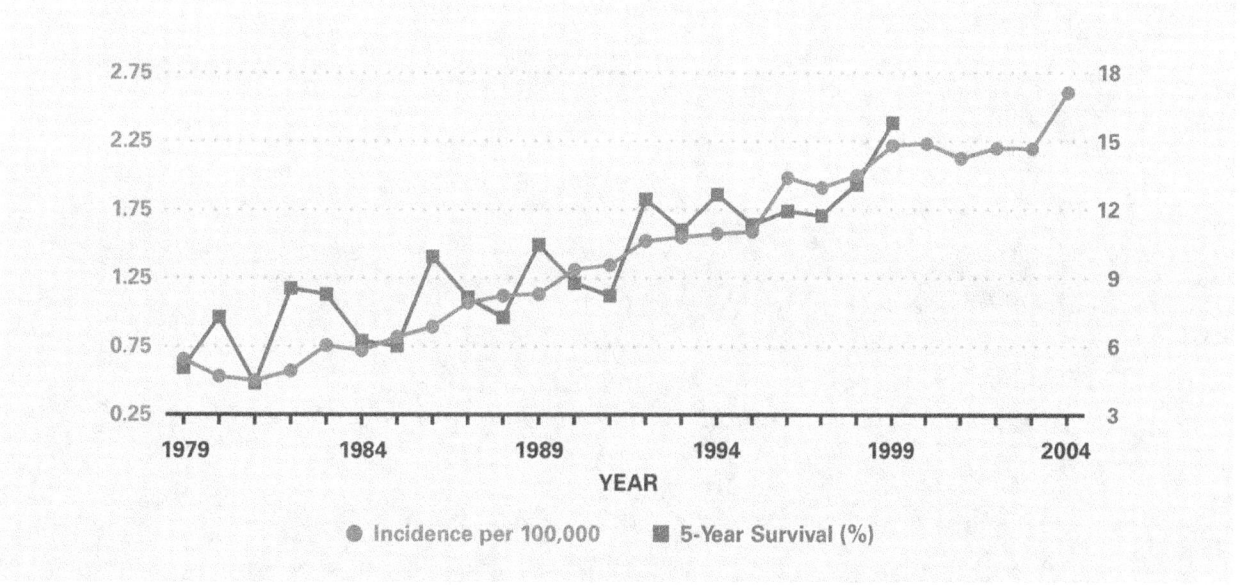

SOURCE: Surveillance, Epidemiology, and End Results (SEER) Program

Table 3. All Esophageal Cancer: Number of Cases and Incidence Rates by Age, Race/Ethnicity, and Sex, 2004

			INCIDENCE PER 100,000	
DEMOGRAPHIC CHARACTERISTICS		Number of Cases	Unadjusted	Age-Adjusted
AGE (Years)	Under 15	—	—	—
	15–44	367	0.3	—
	45–64	4,712	6.7	—
	65+	8,411	24.6	—
RACE/ETHNICITY	Non-Hispanic White	11,572	6.0	5.1
	Non-Hispanic Black	1,394	4.1	5.5
	Hispanic	638	1.6	3.4
	Asian/Pacific Islander	299	2.4	2.9
	American Indian/Alaska Native	—	—	—
SEX	Female	3,186	2.2	2.1
	Male	9,605	6.9	8.1
TOTAL		12,863	4.5	—

SOURCE: Surveillance, Epidemiology, and End Results (SEER) Program

Figure 3. All Esophageal Cancer: Age-Adjusted Incidence Rates and 5-Year Survival Rates, 1979–2004

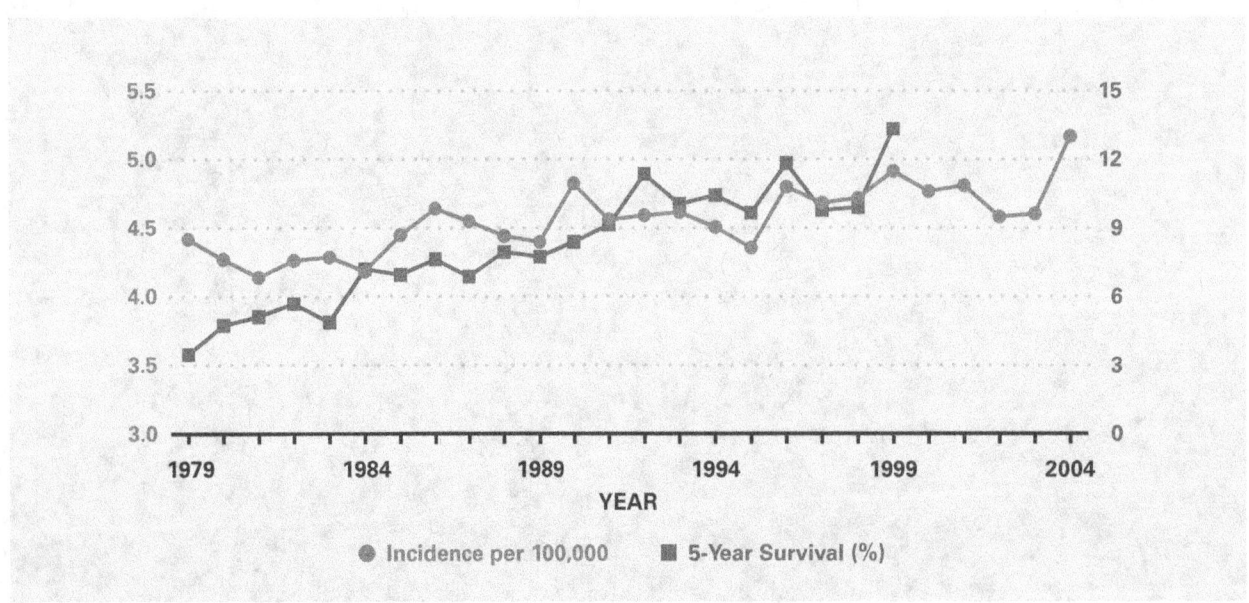

SOURCE: Surveillance, Epidemiology, and End Results (SEER) Program

Table 4. All Esophageal Cancer: Number and Age-Adjusted Rates of Ambulatory Care Visits and Hospital Discharges With First-Listed and All-Listed Diagnoses by Age, Race, and Sex in the United States, 2004

DEMOGRAPHIC CHARACTERISTICS		AMBULATORY CARE VISITS				HOSPITAL DISCHARGES			
		First-Listed Diagnosis		All-Listed Diagnoses		First-Listed Diagnosis		All-Listed Diagnoses	
		Number in Thousands	Rate per 100,000	Number in Thousands	Rate per 100,000	Number in Thousands	Rate per 100,000	Number in Thousands	Rate per 100,000
AGE (Years)	Under 15	—	—	—	—	—	—	—	—
	15–44	—	—	—	—	1	1	2	2
	45–64	215	304	217	308	8	11	17	25
	65+	138	379	150	413	11	30	25	69
RACE	White	343	131	361	139	16	6	36	14
	Black	—	—	—	—	2	8	6	19
SEX	Female	—	—	—	—	5	3	10	6
	Male	244	170	261	184	15	11	34	26
TOTAL		354	120	372	127	20	7	44	15

SOURCE: National Ambulatory Medical Care Survey (NAMCS) and National Hospital Ambulatory Medical Care Survey (NHAMCS) (3-year average, 2003–2005), and Healthcare Cost and Utilization Project Nationwide Inpatient Sample (HCUP NIS)

Figure 4. All Esophageal Cancer: Age-Adjusted Rates of Ambulatory Care Visits and Hospital Discharges With All-Listed Diagnoses in the United States, 1979–2004

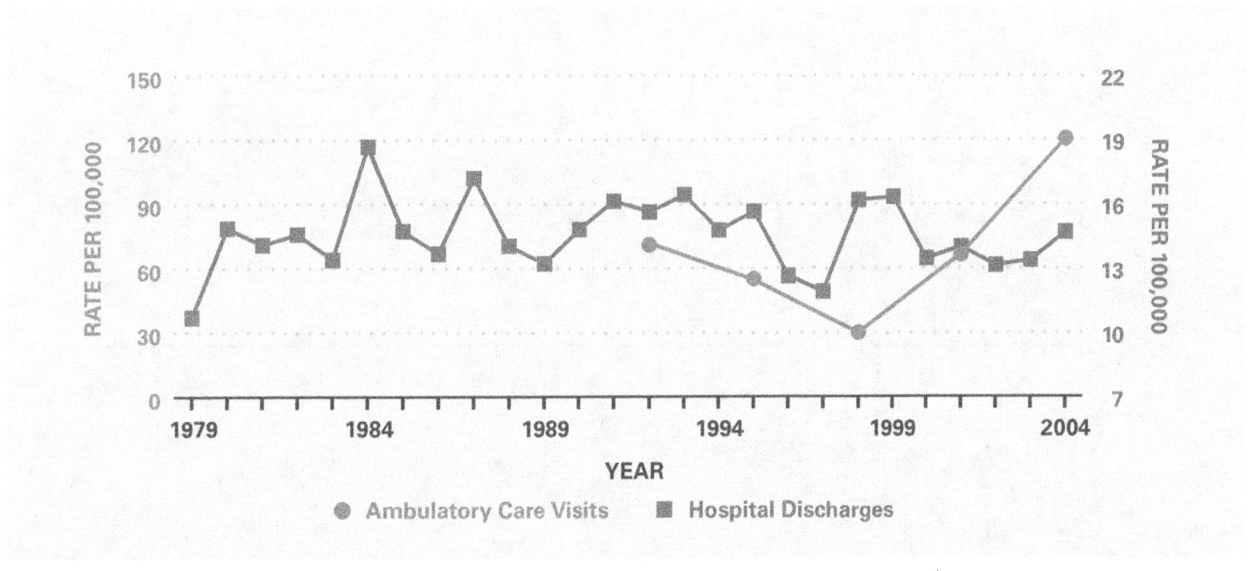

SOURCE: National Ambulatory Medical Care Survey (NAMCS) and National Hospital Ambulatory Medical Care Survey (NHAMCS) (averages 1992–1993, 1994–1996, 1997–1999, 2000–2002, 2003–2005), and National Hospital Discharge Survey (NHDS)

Table 5. All Esophageal Cancer: Number and Age-Adjusted Rates of Deaths and Years of Potential Life Lost (to Age 75) by Age, Race, and Sex in the United States, 2004

DEMOGRAPHIC CHARACTERISTICS		UNDERLYING CAUSE			UNDERLYING OR OTHER CAUSE	
		Number of Deaths	Rate per 100,000	Years of Potential Life Lost in Thousands	Number of Deaths	Rate per 100,000
AGE (Years)	Under 15	—	—	—	—	—
	15–44	371	0.3	12.9	388	0.3
	45–64	4,650	6.6	82.6	4,929	7.0
	65+	8,646	23.8	18.4	9,610	26.4
RACE	White	11,850	4.6	94.6	12,953	5.0
	Black	1,561	5.5	17.0	1,696	6.0
SEX	Female	3,063	1.8	18.5	3,361	2.0
	Male	10,604	8.1	95.4	11,566	8.9
TOTAL		13,667	4.7	113.8	14,927	5.1

SOURCE: Vital Statistics of the United States

Figure 5. All Esophageal Cancer: Age-Adjusted Rates of Death in the United States, 1979–2004

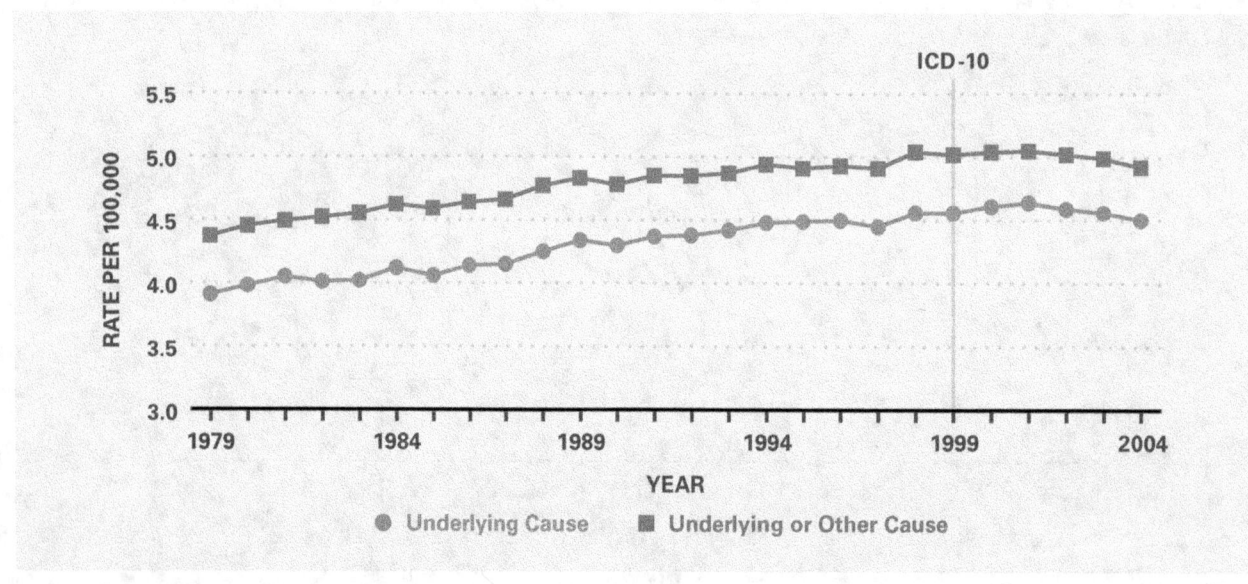

SOURCE: Vital Statistics of the United States

CHAPTER 6

Cancer of the Stomach

James E. Everhart, M.D., M.P.H.

SEER includes cancers of the gastroesophageal junction and gastric cardia with gastric cancer. Over the period 1979 to 2004, the incidence of cancers of the gastroesophageal junction and cardia approximately doubled, resulting in an increase in the proportion of gastric cancer at these sites from 14.9% in 1979 to 30.4% in 2004. However, for medical care and vital statistics, these sites were included with esophageal cancer.

In 2004, the stomach was the third most common anatomical site for digestive system cancer, after the colon/rectum and the pancreas. Cancer of the stomach, gastric cancer, had an older age distribution than did other GI cancers, with 68 percent of cases having occurred at age 65 years or older (Table 1). Median age of diagnosis was 71 years (http://seer.cancer.gov/csr/1975_2005/results_merged/topic_med_age.pdf). Asians and Hispanics had the highest age-adjusted incidence rates; non-Hispanic whites had the lowest rate. The incidence of gastric cancer, as reflected by mortality rates, has been declining for more than 70 years in the United States. Between 1979 and 2004, the incidence declined more than one-third (Figure 1).

During that period, 5-year survival following diagnosis increased by 50 percent.

Ambulatory care visits and hospital discharges with gastric cancer were relatively insubstantial (Table 2). Hospitalization rates declined more rapidly than the incidence rate (Figure 2). Because gastric cancer now has somewhat better survival than other digestive system cancers, it was only the fourth leading cause of death among these cancers. Seventy percent of deaths with gastric cancer as the underlying cause occurred at age 65 years or older (Table 3). The large majority of deaths listed gastric cancer as the underlying cause. Age-adjusted mortality rates were more than twice as high among blacks as whites and nearly twice as high among men as women. If cancer of the gastroesophageal junction were included among gastric cancer, the number of deaths would have increased 5.6 percent to 11,883 in 2004. Reflecting the declining incidence rate and longer survival, the age-adjusted mortality rate of gastric cancer declined by 49 percent between 1979 and 2004 (Figure 3), the most rapid decline for any major digestive system cancer.

Table 1. Gastric Cancer: Number of Cases and Incidence Rates by Age, Race/Ethnicity, and Sex, 2004

DEMOGRAPHIC CHARACTERISTICS		Number of Cases	INCIDENCE PER 100,000	
			Unadjusted	Age-Adjusted
AGE (Years)	Under 15	—	—	—
	15–44	1,292	1.1	—
	45–64	6,610	9.4	—
	65+	14,617	42.7	—
RACE/ETHNICITY	Non-Hispanic White	14,224	7.4	6.2
	Non-Hispanic Black	2,727	8.0	11.4
	Hispanic	2,425	6.0	12.3
	Asian/Pacific Islander	1,419	11.5	13.8
	American Indian/Alaska Native	123	6.6	9.1
SEX	Female	8,579	5.9	5.5
	Male	12,888	9.2	11.1
TOTAL		21,519	7.5	—

SOURCE: Surveillance, Epidemiology, and End Results (SEER) Program

Figure 1. Gastric Cancer: Age-Adjusted Incidence Rates and 5-Year Survival Rates, 1979–2004

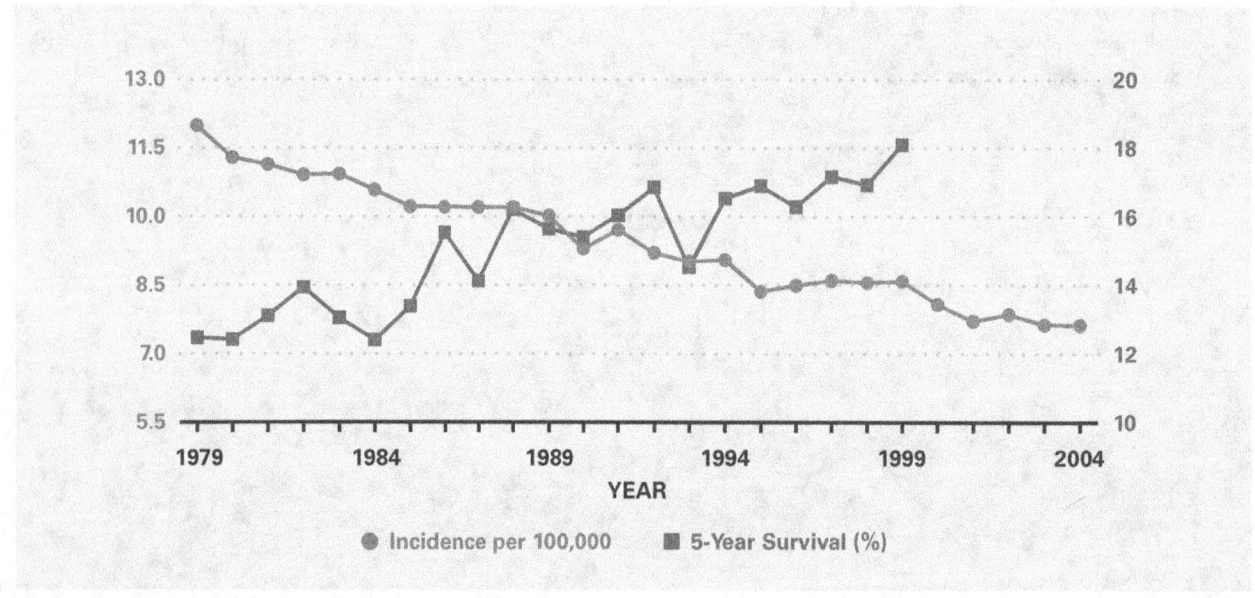

SOURCE: Surveillance, Epidemiology, and End Results (SEER) Program

Table 2. Gastric Cancer: Number and Age-Adjusted Rates of Ambulatory Care Visits and Hospital Discharges With First-Listed and All-Listed Diagnoses by Age, Race, and Sex in the United States, 2004

		AMBULATORY CARE VISITS				HOSPITAL DISCHARGES			
		First-Listed Diagnosis		All-Listed Diagnoses		First-Listed Diagnosis		All-Listed Diagnoses	
DEMOGRAPHIC CHARACTERISTICS		Number in Thousands	Rate per 100,000	Number in Thousands	Rate per 100,000	Number in Thousands	Rate per 100,000	Number in Thousands	Rate per 100,000
AGE (Years)	Under 15	—	—	—	—	—	—	—	—
	15–44	—	—	—	—	1	1	3	2
	45–64	—	—	—	—	5	7	10	14
	65+	—	—	107	295	10	29	19	52
RACE	White	—	—	99	40	11	4	21	8
	Black	—	—	—	—	3	11	6	21
SEX	Female	—	—	—	—	7	4	14	8
	Male	—	—	59	44	9	7	17	13
TOTAL		137	47	141	48	17	6	31	11

SOURCE: National Ambulatory Medical Care Survey (NAMCS) and National Hospital Ambulatory Medical Care Survey (NHAMCS) (3-year average, 2003–2005), and Healthcare Cost and Utilization Project Nationwide Inpatient Sample (HCUP NIS)

Figure 2. Gastric Cancer: Age-Adjusted Rates of Ambulatory Care Visits and Hospital Discharges With All-Listed Diagnoses in the United States, 1979–2004

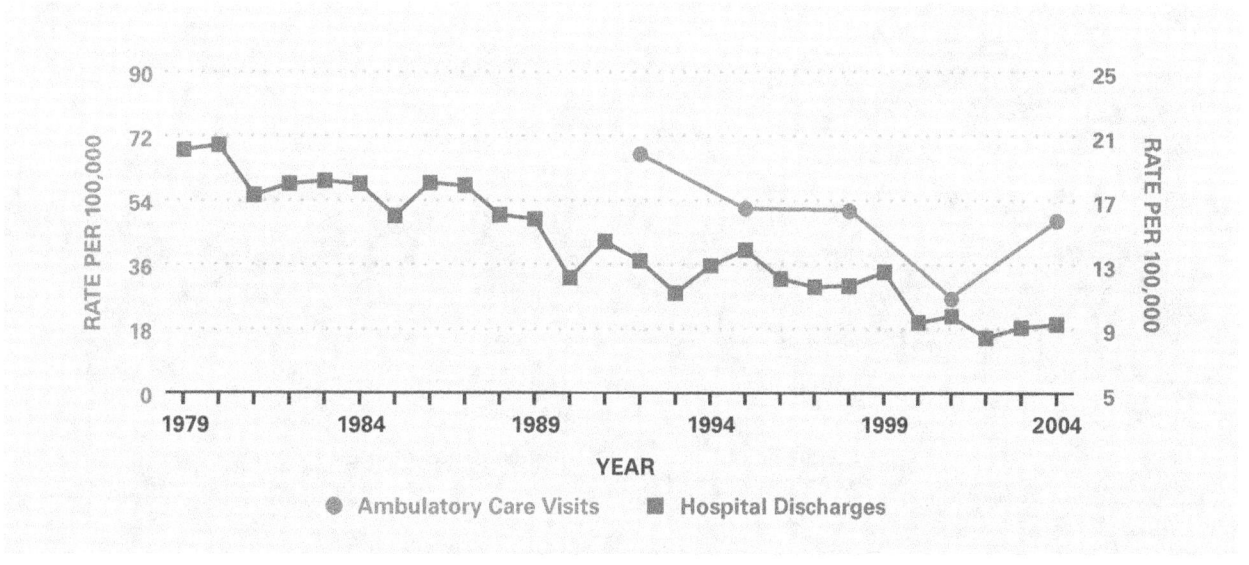

SOURCE: National Ambulatory Medical Care Survey (NAMCS) and National Hospital Ambulatory Medical Care Survey (NHAMCS) (averages 1992–1993, 1994–1996, 1997–1999, 2000–2002, 2003–2005), and National Hospital Discharge Survey (NHDS)

Table 3. Gastric Cancer: Number and Age-Adjusted Rates of Deaths and Years of Potential Life Lost (to Age 75) by Age, Race, and Sex in the United States, 2004

DEMOGRAPHIC CHARACTERISTICS		UNDERLYING CAUSE			UNDERLYING OR OTHER CAUSE	
		Number of Deaths	Rate per 100,000	Years of Potential Life Lost in Thousands	Number of Deaths	Rate per 100,000
AGE (Years)	Under 15	—	—	—	—	—
	15–44	573	0.5	20.7	585	0.5
	45–64	2,809	4.0	51.8	2,942	4.2
	65+	7,871	21.7	11.7	8,734	24.0
RACE	White	8,494	3.3	58.0	9,271	3.6
	Black	2,008	7.5	18.7	2,177	8.1
SEX	Female	4,791	2.8	32.9	5,197	3.0
	Male	6,462	5.2	51.3	7,064	5.7
TOTAL		11,253	3.8	84.2	12,261	4.2

SOURCE: Vital Statistics of the United States

Figure 3. Gastric Cancer: Age-Adjusted Rates of Death in the United States, 1979–2004

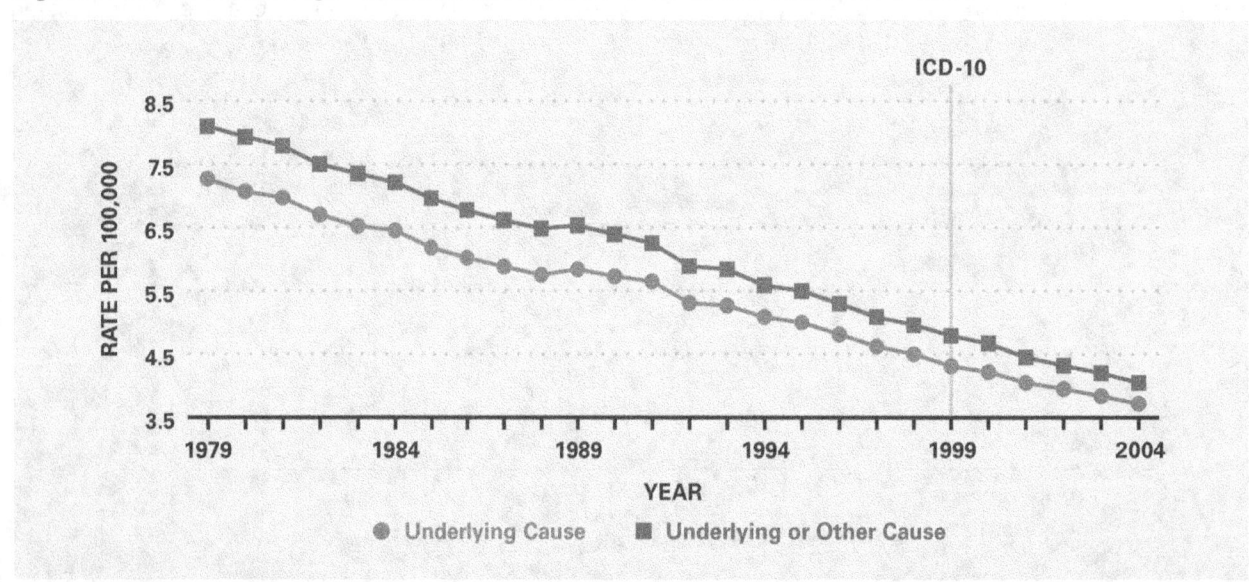

SOURCE: Vital Statistics of the United States

CHAPTER 7

Cancer of the Small Intestine

James E. Everhart, M.D., M.P.H.

Cancer of the small intestine is often considered rare, but in 2004, there were more than 5,000 new cases diagnosed (exclusive of intestinal lymphomas), or about a third the total number of esophageal cancers or primary liver cancers, and more than the number of gallbladder cancers. Slightly more than half of patients were diagnosed at age 65 years or older (Table 1), with a median age of 67 years (http://seer.cancer.gov/csr/1975_2005/results_merged/topic_med_age.pdf), making this the digestive system cancer with the second youngest age of onset (after primary liver cancer). Nevertheless, rates were highest among the elderly and among blacks and males.

Age-adjusted incidence for cancer of the small intestine increased by 73 percent between 1979 and 2004 (Figure 1). Lack of awareness of the magnitude of this increase may be a reason for the perception that

it remains a rare cancer. Over the same period, 5-year survival improved modestly, from about 33 percent to about 41 percent. National medical care systems do not adequately capture outpatient or inpatient visits (Table 2), although rates of hospital discharges have tended to increase in recent years (Figure 2). The number of hospitalizations prior to 1988 was too small to provide estimates.

Because of its relatively high survival rate, there were only 1,115 deaths from cancer of the small intestine in 2004, and fewer than 10,000 YPLL prior to age 75 years (Table 3). The majority of deaths occurred among persons age 65 years and older. Death rates were higher for blacks than whites and for males than females, reflecting the incidence rates. Age-adjusted death rates changed little between 1979 and 2004 (Figure 3).

Table 1. Cancer of the Small Intestine: Number of Cases and Incidence Rates by Age, Race/Ethnicity, and Sex, 2004

DEMOGRAPHIC CHARACTERISTICS		Number of Cases	INCIDENCE PER 100,000	
			Unadjusted	Age-Adjusted
AGE (Years)	Under 15	—	—	—
	15–44	407	0.3	—
	45–64	1,987	2.8	—
	65+	2,889	8.4	—
RACE/ETHNICITY	Non-Hispanic White	4,298	2.2	1.9
	Non-Hispanic Black	756	2.2	3.0
	Hispanic	295	0.7	1.4
	Asian/Pacific Islander	107	0.9	1.0
	American Indian/Alaska Native	—	—	—
SEX	Female	2,357	1.6	1.5
	Male	2,703	1.9	2.2
TOTAL		5,065	1.8	—

SOURCE: Surveillance, Epidemiology, and End Results (SEER) Program

Figure 1. Cancer of the Small Intestine: Age-Adjusted Incidence Rates and 5-Year Survival Rates, 1979–2004

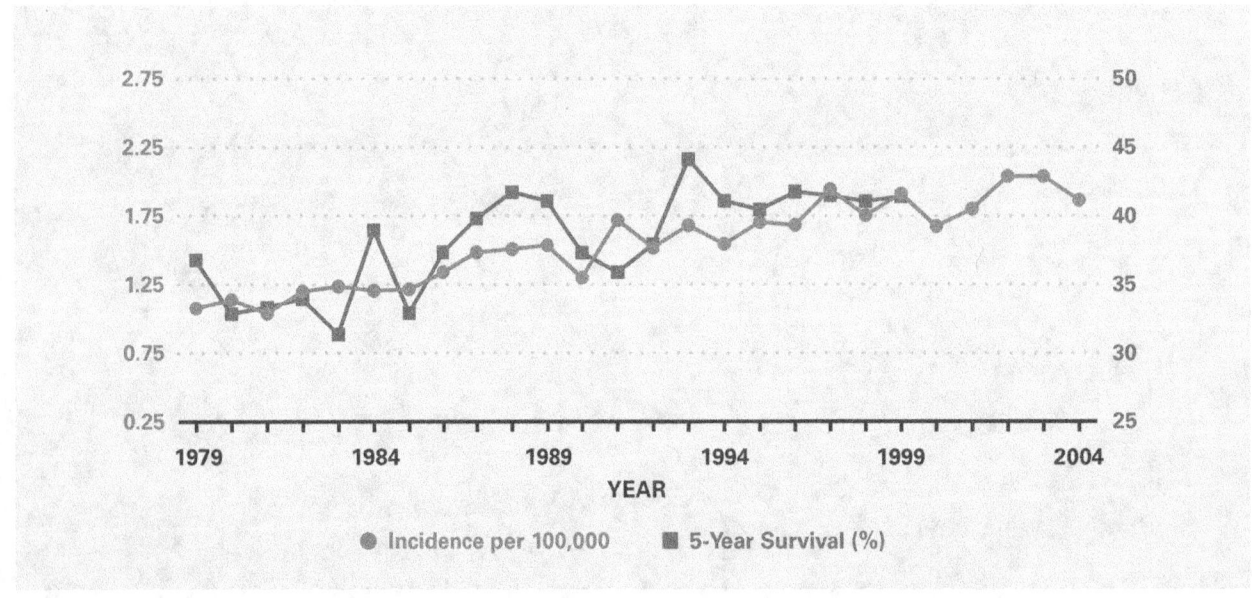

SOURCE: Surveillance, Epidemiology, and End Results (SEER) Program

Table 2. Cancer of the Small Intestine: Number and Age-Adjusted Rates of Ambulatory Care Visits and Hospital Discharges With First-Listed and All-Listed Diagnoses by Age, Race, and Sex in the United States, 2004

DEMOGRAPHIC CHARACTERISTICS		AMBULATORY CARE VISITS				HOSPITAL DISCHARGES			
		First-Listed Diagnosis		All-Listed Diagnoses		First-Listed Diagnosis		All-Listed Diagnoses	
		Number in Thousands	Rate per 100,000	Number in Thousands	Rate per 100,000	Number in Thousands	Rate per 100,000	Number in Thousands	Rate per 100,000
AGE (Years)	Under 15	—	—	—	—	—	—	—	—
	15–44	—	—	—	—	0	0	1	1
	45–64	—	—	—	—	2	3	3	5
	65+	—	—	—	—	3	9	5	14
RACE	White	—	—	—	—	5	2	7	3
	Black	—	—	—	—	1	3	1	5
SEX	Female	—	—	—	—	3	2	4	3
	Male	—	—	—	—	3	2	5	4
TOTAL		—	—	—	—	6	2	9	3

SOURCE: National Ambulatory Medical Care Survey (NAMCS) and National Hospital Ambulatory Medical Care Survey (NHAMCS) (3-year average, 2003–2005), and Healthcare Cost and Utilization Project Nationwide Inpatient Sample (HCUP NIS)

Figure 2. Cancer of the Small Intestine: Age-Adjusted Rates of Ambulatory Care Visits and Hospital Discharges With All-Listed Diagnoses in the United States, 1979–2004 (Ambulatory Care Visit Data Unavailable)

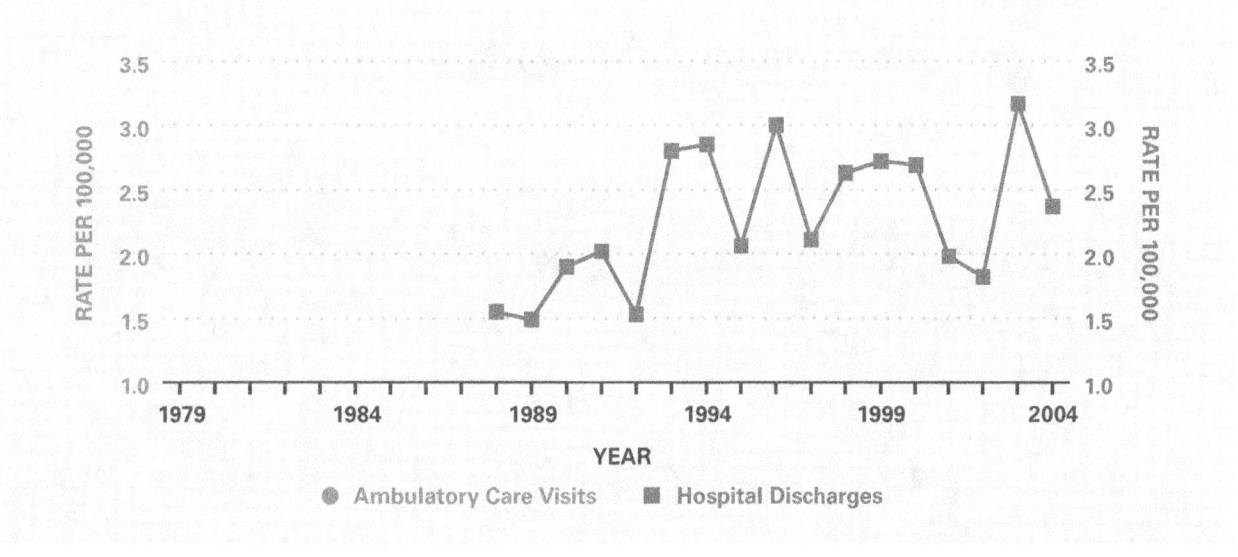

SOURCE: National Ambulatory Medical Care Survey (NAMCS) and National Hospital Ambulatory Medical Care Survey (NHAMCS) (averages 1992–1993, 1994–1996, 1997–1999, 2000–2002, 2003–2005), and National Hospital Discharge Survey (NHDS)

Table 3. Cancer of the Small Intestine: Number and Age-Adjusted Rates of Deaths and Years of Potential Life Lost (to Age 75) by Age, Race, and Sex in the United States, 2004

DEMOGRAPHIC CHARACTERISTICS		UNDERLYING CAUSE			UNDERLYING OR OTHER CAUSE	
		Number of Deaths	Rate per 100,000	Years of Potential Life Lost in Thousands	Number of Deaths	Rate per 100,000
AGE (Years)	Under 15	—	—	—	—	—
	15–44	55	0.0	2.0	59	0.0
	45–64	329	0.5	6.0	358	0.5
	65+	731	2.0	1.4	838	2.3
RACE	White	908	0.3	6.9	1,021	0.4
	Black	175	0.6	2.1	194	0.7
SEX	Female	523	0.3	4.3	588	0.3
	Male	592	0.5	5.0	667	0.5
TOTAL		1,115	0.4	9.3	1,255	0.4

SOURCE: Vital Statistics of the United States

Figure 3. Cancer of the Small Intestine: Age-Adjusted Rates of Death in the United States, 1979–2004

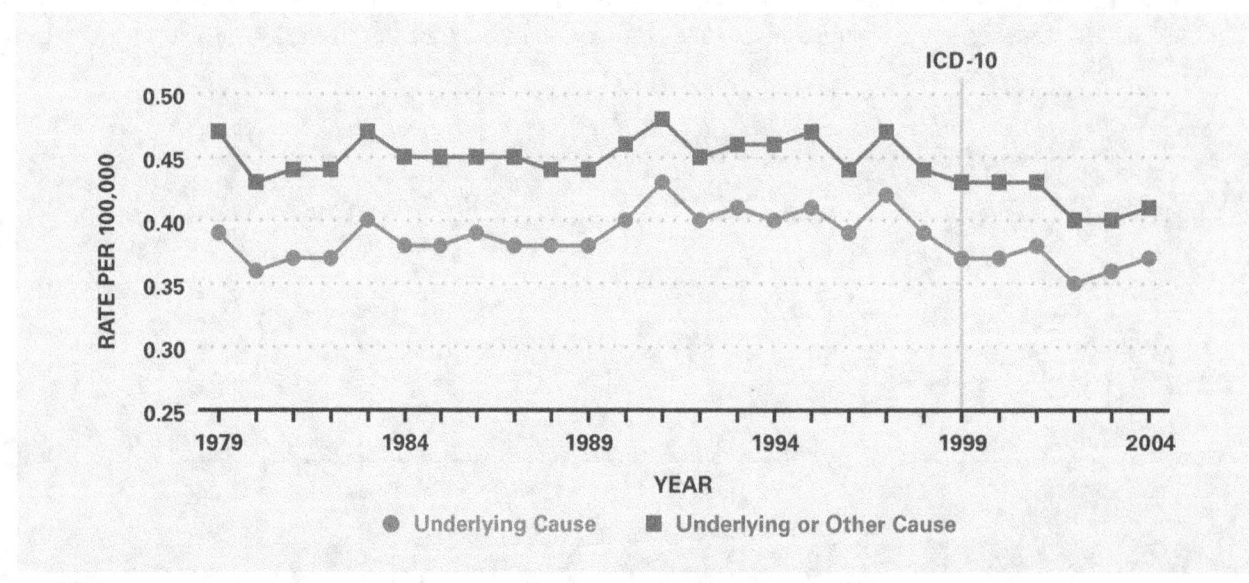

SOURCE: Vital Statistics of the United States

CHAPTER 8

Cancer of the Colon and Rectum

James E. Everhart, M.D., M.P.H.

For this report, cancers of the colon and rectum were combined (see Appendix 1 for ICD codes). Together, these cancers were responsible for an estimated 55 percent of all digestive system cancers diagnosed in 2004. In 72.5 percent of cases, the colon was the anatomical site. By themselves, colon cancer would be the most common digestive system cancer, and rectal cancer the second most common. Therefore, trends in colorectal cancer largely determine trends in digestive system cancers as a whole.

Two-thirds of new cases of colorectal cancer were among those age 65 years or older (Table 1). Among the major racial-ethnic groups, non-Hispanic blacks had the highest rate, followed by non-Hispanic whites. American Indians had the lowest rates, with Hispanics and Asians intermediate. Age-adjusted rates were about one-third higher among males than females. Colorectal cancer incidence has been falling for the past 20 years, declining by 27.1 percent from 1985 to 2004 (Figure 1). The proportion of newly diagnosed patients who survived for at least 5 years has climbed steadily since 1979.

Colorectal cancer is the digestive system malignancy with the most reliable data on medical care (Table 2). In 2004, there were an estimated 2.6 million ambulatory care visits for persons with colorectal cancer. Most visits were among persons age 65 years and older and among women. Blacks had two-thirds the age-adjusted rate of whites. Visit rates were similar for males and females. For hospitalizations, colorectal cancer was more often listed as a first-listed diagnosis than as a secondary diagnosis. Hospitalization rates were disproportionately higher among the 65 years and older group. Age-adjusted rates were higher for blacks than for whites and for males than for females. Hospitalization rates declined from the early 1980s through 1995, and subsequently increased slightly (Figure 2).

Colorectal cancer was the leading cause of death related to the digestive system, accounting for 22.5 percent of deaths (Table 3). Because the median age of death for colorectal cancer was 75 years (http://seer.cancer.gov/csr/1975_2005/results_merged/topic_med_age.pdf), colorectal cancer accounted for a smaller proportion of YPLL to digestive diseases (16.6 percent), second to liver disease. Because of declining incidence and improved survival, death rates declined 34.8 percent between 1979 and 2004. This decline accelerated during the latter part of that period (Figure 3).

Table 1. Colorectal Cancer: Number of Cases and Incidence Rates by Age, Race/Ethnicity, and Sex, 2004

			INCIDENCE PER 100,000	
DEMOGRAPHIC CHARACTERISTICS		Number of Cases	Unadjusted	Age-Adjusted
AGE (Years)	Under 15	—	—	—
	15–44	6,019	5.0	—
	45–64	41,467	59.2	—
	65+	87,872	256.9	—
RACE/ETHNICITY	Non-Hispanic White	111,509	58.0	48.5
	Non-Hispanic Black	14,251	41.7	58.6
	Hispanic	7,370	18.2	38.1
	Asian/Pacific Islander	4,089	33.2	38.6
	American Indian/Alaska Native	477	25.8	35.8
SEX	Female	64,080	43.9	41.1
	Male	65,069	46.5	55.7
TOTAL		129,189	45.2	47.5

SOURCE: Surveillance, Epidemiology, and End Results (SEER) Program

Figure 1. Colorectal Cancer: Age-Adjusted Incidence Rates and 5-Year Survival Rates, 1979–2004

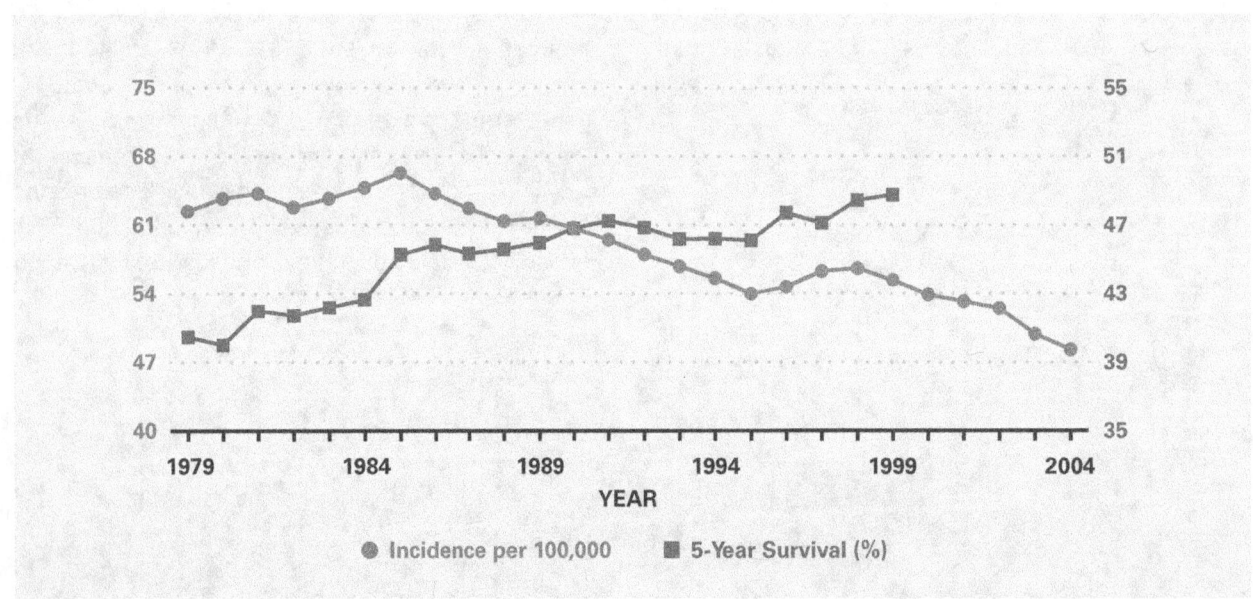

SOURCE: Surveillance, Epidemiology, and End Results (SEER) Program

Table 2. Colorectal Cancer: Number and Age-Adjusted Rates of Ambulatory Care Visits and Hospital Discharges With First-Listed and All-Listed Diagnoses by Age, Race, and Sex in the United States, 2004

DEMOGRAPHIC CHARACTERISTICS		AMBULATORY CARE VISITS				HOSPITAL DISCHARGES			
		First-Listed Diagnosis		All-Listed Diagnoses		First-Listed Diagnosis		All-Listed Diagnoses	
		Number in Thousands	Rate per 100,000	Number in Thousands	Rate per 100,000	Number in Thousands	Rate per 100,000	Number in Thousands	Rate per 100,000
AGE (Years)	Under 15	—	—	—	—	—	—	—	—
	15–44	56	45	83	66	7	6	14	11
	45–64	721	1,021	875	1,238	47	66	80	113
	65+	1,321	3,636	1,627	4,477	97	268	160	441
RACE	White	1,892	747	2,323	915	118	45	195	76
	Black	127	426	177	601	17	59	30	107
SEX	Female	1,134	705	1,456	902	76	45	127	75
	Male	969	736	1,133	856	76	58	127	98
TOTAL		2,103	716	2,589	882	151	52	255	87

SOURCE: National Ambulatory Medical Care Survey (NAMCS) and National Hospital Ambulatory Medical Care Survey (NHAMCS) (3-year average, 2003–2005), and Healthcare Cost and Utilization Project Nationwide Inpatient Sample (HCUP NIS)

Figure 2. Colorectal Cancer: Age-Adjusted Rates of Ambulatory Care Visits and Hospital Discharges With All-Listed Diagnoses in the United States, 1979–2004

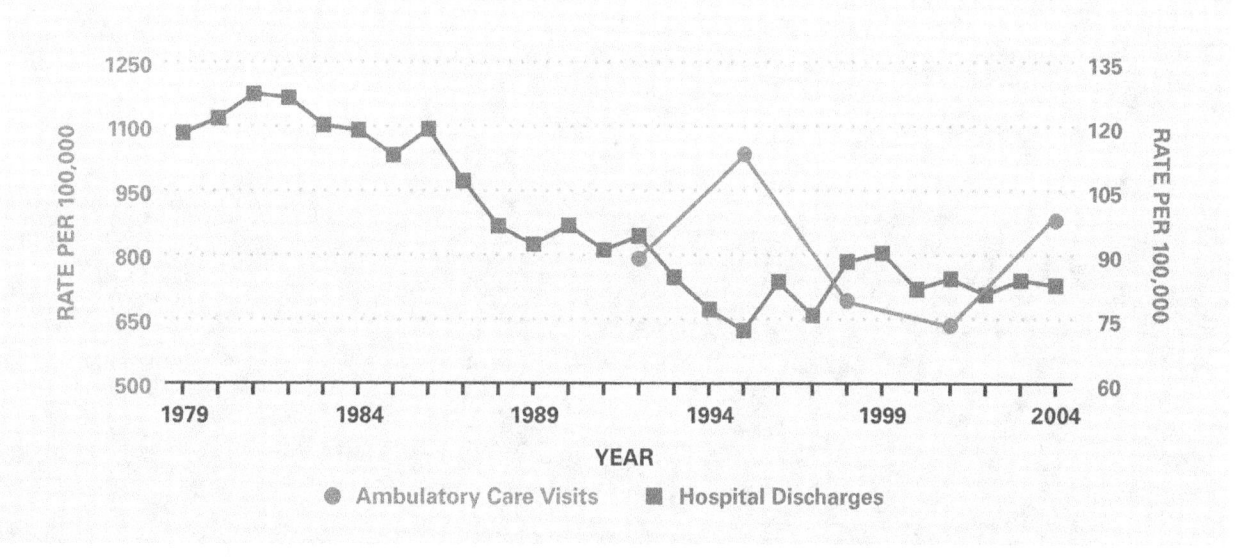

SOURCE: National Ambulatory Medical Care Survey (NAMCS) and National Hospital Ambulatory Medical Care Survey (NHAMCS) (averages 1992–1993, 1994–1996, 1997–1999, 2000–2002, 2003–2005), and National Hospital Discharge Survey (NHDS)

Table 3. Colorectal Cancer: Number and Age-Adjusted Rates of Deaths and Years of Potential Life Lost (to Age 75) by Age, Race, and Sex in the United States, 2004

DEMOGRAPHIC CHARACTERISTICS		UNDERLYING CAUSE			UNDERLYING OR OTHER CAUSE	
		Number of Deaths	Rate per 100,000	Years of Potential Life Lost in Thousands	Number of Deaths	Rate per 100,000
AGE (Years)	Under 15	1	0.0	0.1	2	0.0
	15–44	1,608	1.3	58.3	1,654	1.3
	45–64	12,262	17.3	219.9	13,056	18.5
	65+	39,355	108.3	54.9	48,188	132.6
RACE	White	45,340	17.3	263.0	53,979	20.6
	Black	6,592	24.7	57.7	7,446	28.2
SEX	Female	26,512	15.1	142.8	31,153	17.5
	Male	26,714	21.5	190.2	31,747	25.9
TOTAL		53,226	18.1	333.0	62,900	21.4

SOURCE: Vital Statistics of the United States

Figure 3. Colorectal Cancer: Age-Adjusted Rates of Death in the United States, 1979–2004

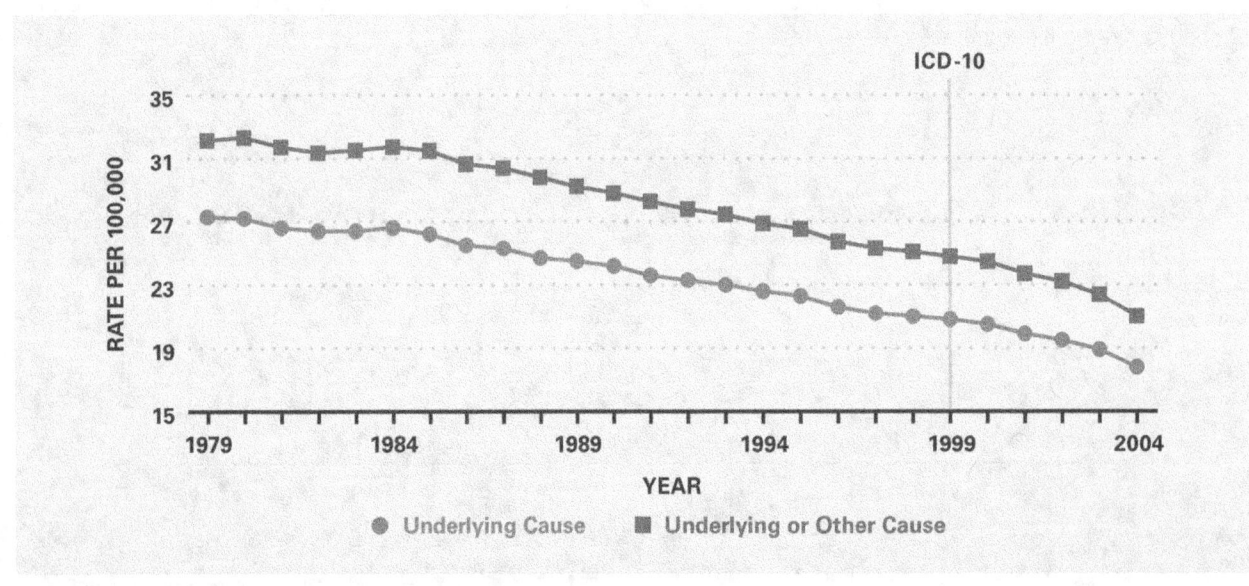

SOURCE: Vital Statistics of the United States

CHAPTER 9

Primary Liver Cancer

James E. Everhart, M.D., M.P.H.

The major malignant neoplasm of the liver is liver cell cancer (hepatocellular carcinoma). Also included in this category in this report are the rare malignancies of hepatoblastoma and angiosarcoma as well as other primary specified and unspecified liver carcinomas. Intrahepatic bile duct carcinoma is included among bile duct cancers (see Appendix 1 for ICD codes).

In 2004, primary liver cancer occurred at an earlier age than any other digestive system cancer, with 50 percent of cases being diagnosed under the age of 65 years (Table 1). Hepatoblastoma, although the most common liver neoplasm among children, had minimal influence on this association because of its rarity. Incidence was lowest among non-Hispanic whites, intermediate among non-Hispanic blacks and Hispanics, and highest among Asians and American Indians. Males had more than 3 times the age-adjusted incidence of females.

The incidence of primary liver cancer rose modestly between 1979 and 1988 (14.5 percent) and more rapidly subsequently (90 percent over the period 1988–2004) (Figure 1). Liver cancer was one of the most lethal digestive system cancers, although 5-year survival did increase nearly fourfold during this period, albeit to only 8 percent.

Medical care visits and hospitalizations for liver cancer were too infrequent in 2004 to make firm statements about them. Hospitalization discharge rates (Table 2) had a demographic pattern similar to incidence rates (Table 1), with the highest rates among patients age 65 years and older, blacks, and males. Hospitalization rates more than doubled from 1984 to 2004 (Figure 2), also in keeping with the increase in incidence.

Death rates increased with age, but not as markedly as in other digestive system cancers (Table 3). Age-adjusted death rates were higher among blacks and males. Because of its increasing incidence and poor survival, primary liver cancer has contributed an increasing number and proportion of deaths, although it accounted for only 4.7 percent of all deaths from digestive system cancers in 2004. Because of the relatively early age of onset, it accounted for a higher proportion of YPLL due to digestive system cancers (7.7 percent). As with incidence, mortality rate increased, although not as quickly. The mortality rate increased 75 percent between 1979 and 2004 (Figure 3).

Table 1. Primary Liver Cancer: Number of Cases and Incidence Rates by Age, Race/Ethnicity, and Sex, 2004

DEMOGRAPHIC CHARACTERISTICS		Number of Cases	INCIDENCE PER 100,000	
			Unadjusted	Age-Adjusted
AGE (Years)	Under 15	165	0.3	—
	15–44	856	0.7	—
	45–64	7,863	11.2	—
	65+	8,093	23.7	—
RACE/ETHNICITY	Non-Hispanic White	9,507	4.9	4.2
	Non-Hispanic Black	2,244	6.6	8.3
	Hispanic	1,894	4.7	9.0
	Asian/Pacific Islander	1,414	11.5	12.9
	American Indian/Alaska Native	151	8.2	10.0
SEX	Female	4,350	3.0	2.8
	Male	11,827	8.5	9.4
TOTAL		16,260	5.7	—

SOURCE: Surveillance, Epidemiology, and End Results (SEER) Program

Figure 1. Primary Liver Cancer: Age-Adjusted Incidence Rates and 5-Year Survival Rates, 1979–2004

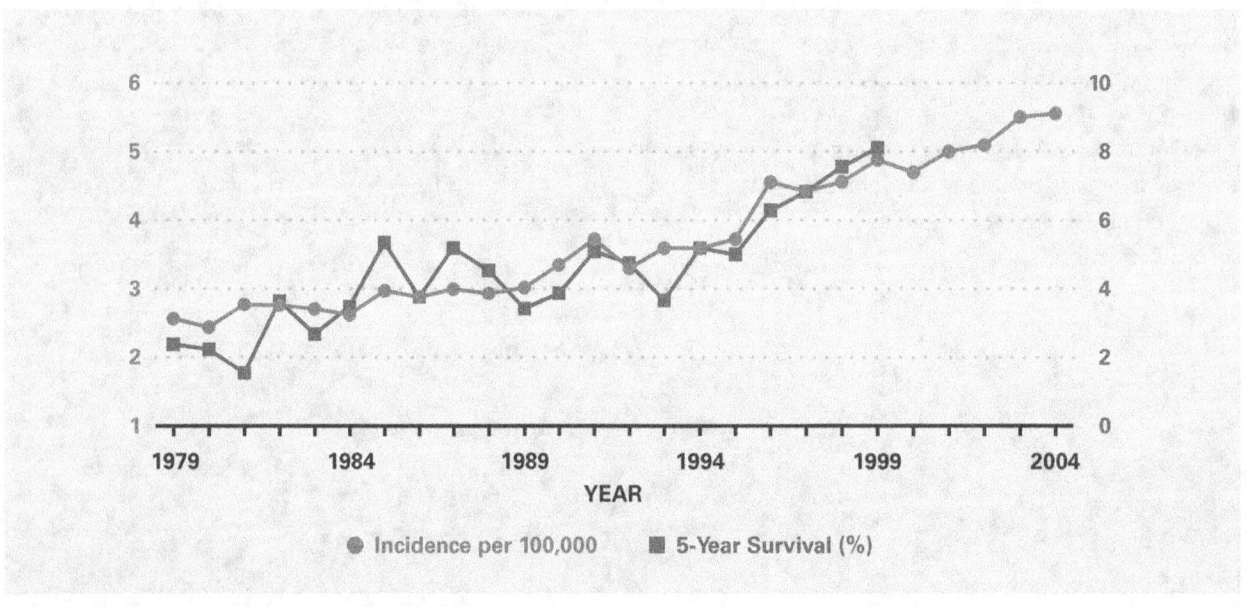

SOURCE: Surveillance, Epidemiology, and End Results (SEER) Program

Table 2. Primary Liver Cancer: Number and Age-Adjusted Rates of Ambulatory Care Visits and Hospital Discharges With First-Listed and All-Listed Diagnoses by Age, Race, and Sex in the United States, 2004

DEMOGRAPHIC CHARACTERISTICS		AMBULATORY CARE VISITS				HOSPITAL DISCHARGES			
		First-Listed Diagnosis		All-Listed Diagnoses		First-Listed Diagnosis		All-Listed Diagnoses	
		Number in Thousands	Rate per 100,000	Number in Thousands	Rate per 100,000	Number in Thousands	Rate per 100,000	Number in Thousands	Rate per 100,000
AGE (Years)	Under 15	—	—	—	—	0	1	2	3
	15–44	—	—	—	—	1	1	2	2
	45–64	—	—	—	—	6	9	15	21
	65+	—	—	—	—	6	17	14	39
RACE	White	—	—	—	—	10	4	25	10
	Black	—	—	—	—	2	7	5	14
SEX	Female	—	—	—	—	4	3	9	6
	Male	—	—	—	—	10	7	23	17
TOTAL		—	—	63	21	14	5	33	11

SOURCE: National Ambulatory Medical Care Survey (NAMCS) and National Hospital Ambulatory Medical Care Survey (NHAMCS) (3-year average, 2003–2005), and Healthcare Cost and Utilization Project Nationwide Inpatient Sample (HCUP NIS)

Figure 2. Primary Liver Cancer: Age-Adjusted Rates of Ambulatory Care Visits and Hospital Discharges With All-Listed Diagnoses in the United States, 1979–2004

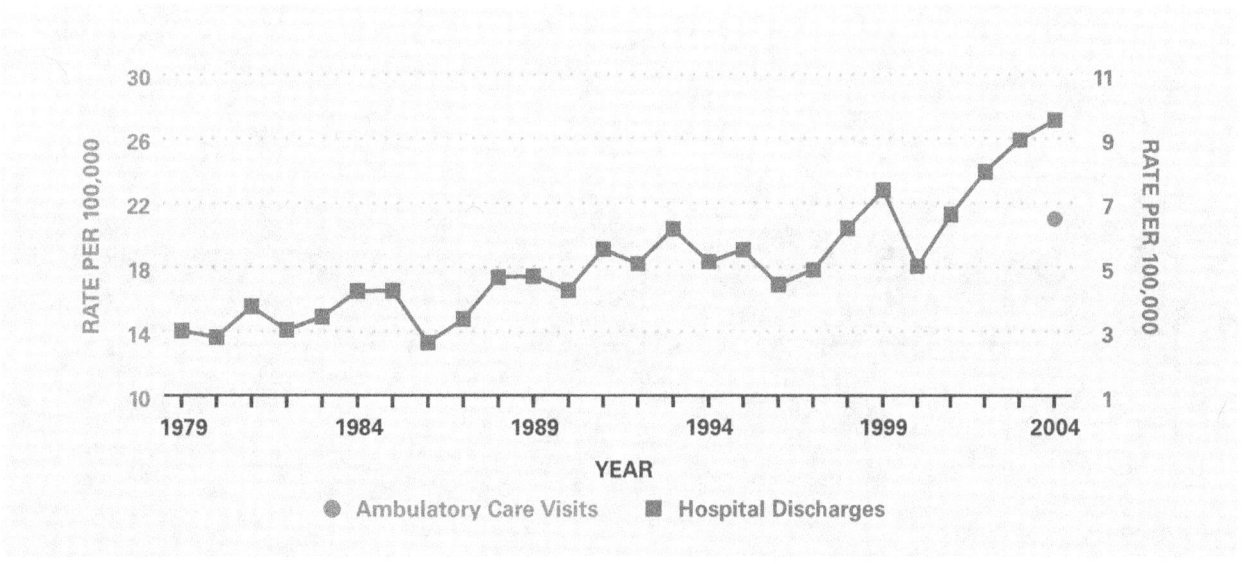

SOURCE: National Ambulatory Medical Care Survey (NAMCS) and National Hospital Ambulatory Medical Care Survey (NHAMCS) (averages 1992–1993, 1994–1996, 1997–1999, 2000–2002, 2003–2005), and National Hospital Discharge Survey (NHDS)

Table 3. Primary Liver Cancer: Number and Age-Adjusted Rates of Deaths and Years of Potential Life Lost (to Age 75) by Age, Race, and Sex in the United States, 2004

DEMOGRAPHIC CHARACTERISTICS		UNDERLYING CAUSE			UNDERLYING OR OTHER CAUSE	
		Number of Deaths	Rate per 100,000	Years of Potential Life Lost in Thousands	Number of Deaths	Rate per 100,000
AGE (Years)	Under 15	33	0.1	2.3	34	0.1
	15–44	243	0.2	9.1	250	0.2
	45–64	2,781	3.9	53.9	3,069	4.3
	65+	3,266	9.0	7.2	3,567	9.8
RACE	White	4,742	1.8	49.8	5,204	2.0
	Black	944	3.1	14.7	1,021	3.4
SEX	Female	1,522	0.9	12.0	1,666	1.0
	Male	4,801	3.5	60.4	5,254	3.9
TOTAL		6,323	2.2	72.4	6,920	2.4

SOURCE: Vital Statistics of the United States

Figure 3. Primary Liver Cancer: Age-Adjusted Rates of Death in the United States, 1979–2004

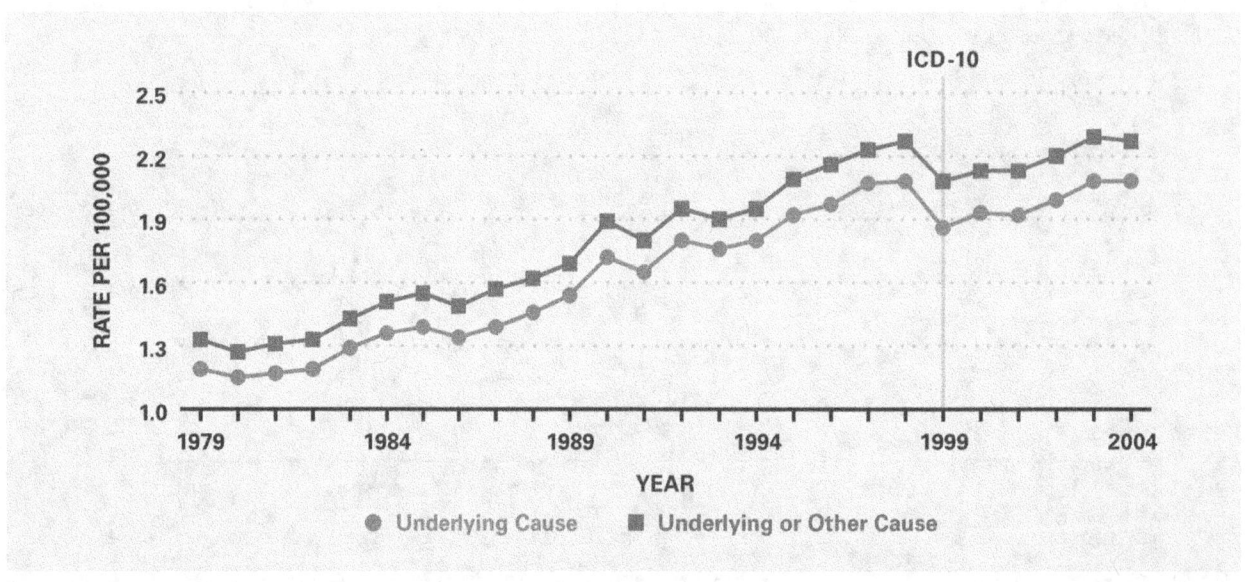

SOURCE: Vital Statistics of the United States

CHAPTER 10

Cancer of the Bile Ducts

James E. Everhart, M.D., M.P.H.

For this report, intrahepatic and extrahepatic bile duct cancers were combined (see Appendix 1 for ICD-9 and ICD-10 codes). Substantial differences between them are noted.

In 2004, 22 percent of bile duct cancer was coded intrahepatic and 45 percent extrahepatic; nearly all the remainder did not have a location specified. Rates were much higher in the oldest age group, with 74 percent of cases occurring at age 65 or older. Age-adjusted rates were highest among Hispanics and Asians (Table 1). Males had a higher rate and slightly higher number of cases than females. Incidence increased modestly between 1979 and 2004 (about 22 percent), all of which could be accounted for by an increase in the incidence of intrahepatic bile duct cancer. Five-year survival did not improve and was about 10 percent for the entire period (Figure 1). There were too few outpatient or inpatient diagnoses to draw inferences about medical care (Table 2), but hospitalization rates were relatively constant at about 5 per 100,000 U.S. population (Figure 2).

Because of low survival, bile duct cancer mortality was similar to incidence. As underlying cause, there were 4,954 deaths in 2004 and nearly 33,000 YPLL prior to age 75 years (Table 3). Rates were highest in the oldest age group. Age-adjusted mortality rates were slightly higher for whites and for males. Death rates for bile duct cancer rose 39 percent between 1979 and 2004 (Figure 3).

Table 1. Bile Duct Cancer: Number of Cases and Incidence Rates by Age, Race/Ethnicity, and Sex, 2004

DEMOGRAPHIC CHARACTERISTICS		Number of Cases	INCIDENCE PER 100,000	
			Unadjusted	Age-Adjusted
AGE (Years)	Under 15	—	—	—
	15–44	266	0.2	—
	45–64	1,655	2.4	—
	65+	4,569	13.4	—
RACE/ETHNICITY	Non-Hispanic White	4,859	2.5	2.1
	Non-Hispanic Black	523	1.5	2.1
	Hispanic	519	1.3	2.8
	Asian/Pacific Islander	332	2.7	3.3
	American Indian/Alaska Native	—	—	—
SEX	Female	3,051	2.1	2.0
	Male	3,133	2.2	2.7
TOTAL		6,186	2.2	—

SOURCE: Surveillance, Epidemiology, and End Results (SEER) Program

Figure 1. Bile Duct Cancer: Age-Adjusted Incidence Rates and 5-Year Survival Rates, 1979–2004

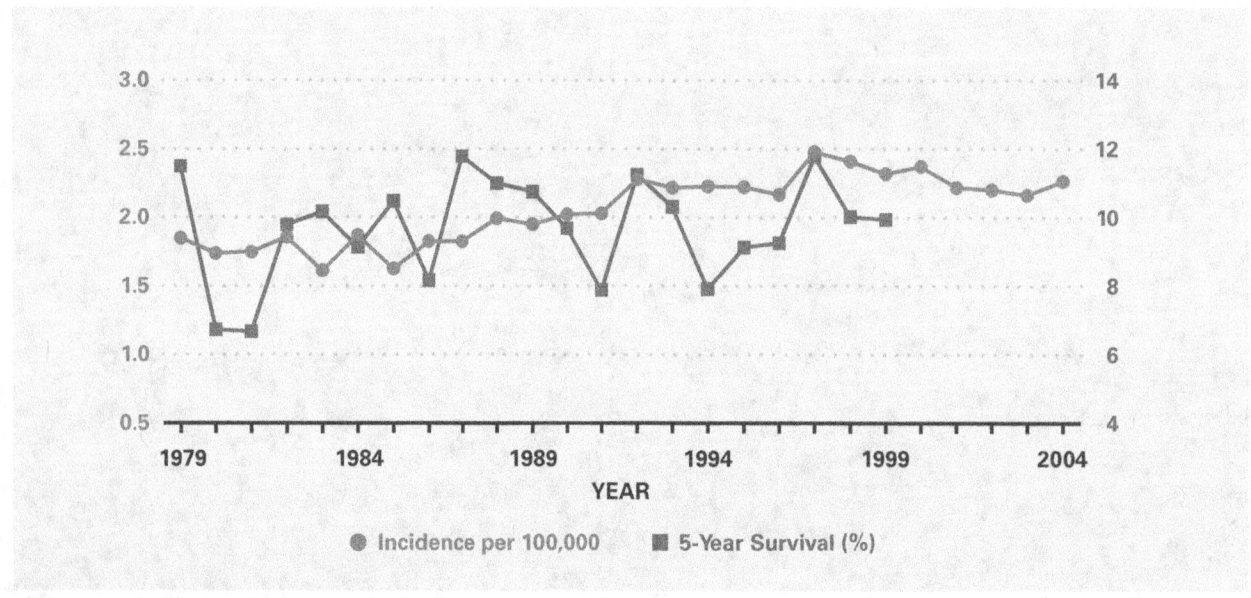

SOURCE: Surveillance, Epidemiology, and End Results (SEER) Program

Table 2. Bile Duct Cancer: Number and Age-Adjusted Rates of Ambulatory Care Visits and Hospital Discharges With First-Listed and All-Listed Diagnoses by Age, Race, and Sex in the United States, 2004

		AMBULATORY CARE VISITS				HOSPITAL DISCHARGES			
		First-Listed Diagnosis		All-Listed Diagnoses		First-Listed Diagnosis		All-Listed Diagnoses	
DEMOGRAPHIC CHARACTERISTICS		Number in Thousands	Rate per 100,000	Number in Thousands	Rate per 100,000	Number in Thousands	Rate per 100,000	Number in Thousands	Rate per 100,000
AGE (Years)	Under 15	—	—	—	—	—	—	—	—
	15–44	—	—	—	—	0	0	1	1
	45–64	—	—	—	—	2	3	5	7
	65+	—	—	—	—	6	17	11	30
RACE	White	—	—	—	—	7	3	14	5
	Black	—	—	—	—	1	3	1	5
SEX	Female	—	—	—	—	4	3	8	5
	Male	—	—	—	—	5	4	9	7
TOTAL		—	—	—	—	9	3	17	6

SOURCE: National Ambulatory Medical Care Survey (NAMCS) and National Hospital Ambulatory Medical Care Survey (NHAMCS) (3-year average, 2003–2005), and Healthcare Cost and Utilization Project Nationwide Inpatient Sample (HCUP NIS)

Figure 2. Bile Duct Cancer: Age-Adjusted Rates of Ambulatory Care Visits and Hospital Discharges With All-Listed Diagnoses in the United States, 1979–2004 (Ambulatory Care Visit Data Unavailable)

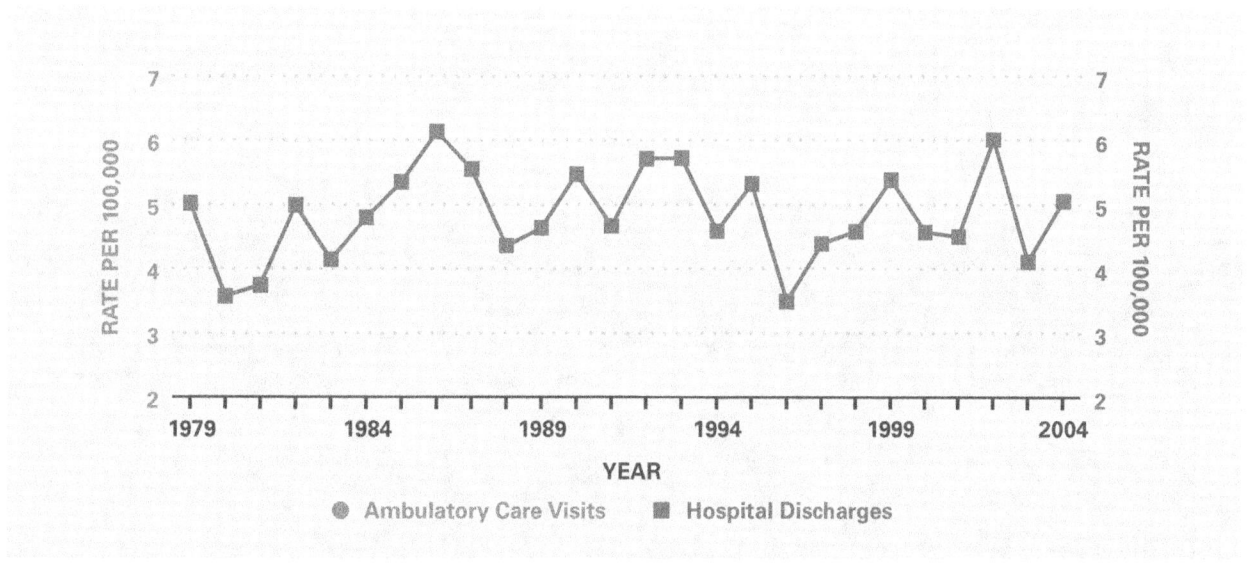

SOURCE: National Ambulatory Medical Care Survey (NAMCS) and National Hospital Ambulatory Medical Care Survey (NHAMCS) (averages 1992–1993, 1994–1996, 1997–1999, 2000–2002, 2003–2005), and National Hospital Discharge Survey (NHDS)

Table 3. Bile Duct Cancer: Number and Age-Adjusted Rates of Deaths and Years of Potential Life Lost (to Age 75) by Age, Race, and Sex in the United States, 2004

DEMOGRAPHIC CHARACTERISTICS		UNDERLYING CAUSE			UNDERLYING OR OTHER CAUSE	
		Number of Deaths	Rate per 100,000	Years of Potential Life Lost in Thousands	Number of Deaths	Rate per 100,000
AGE (Years)	Under 15	2	0.0	0.1	3	0.0
	15–44	143	0.1	5.2	148	0.1
	45–64	1,245	1.8	21.9	1,308	1.9
	65+	3,564	9.8	5.7	3,855	10.6
RACE	White	4,348	1.7	27.6	4,657	1.8
	Black	366	1.4	3.4	401	1.5
SEX	Female	2,554	1.5	15.1	2,711	1.6
	Male	2,400	1.9	17.8	2,603	2.1
TOTAL		4,954	1.7	32.9	5,314	1.8

SOURCE: Vital Statistics of the United States

Figure 3. Bile Duct Cancer: Age-Adjusted Rates of Death in the United States, 1979–2004

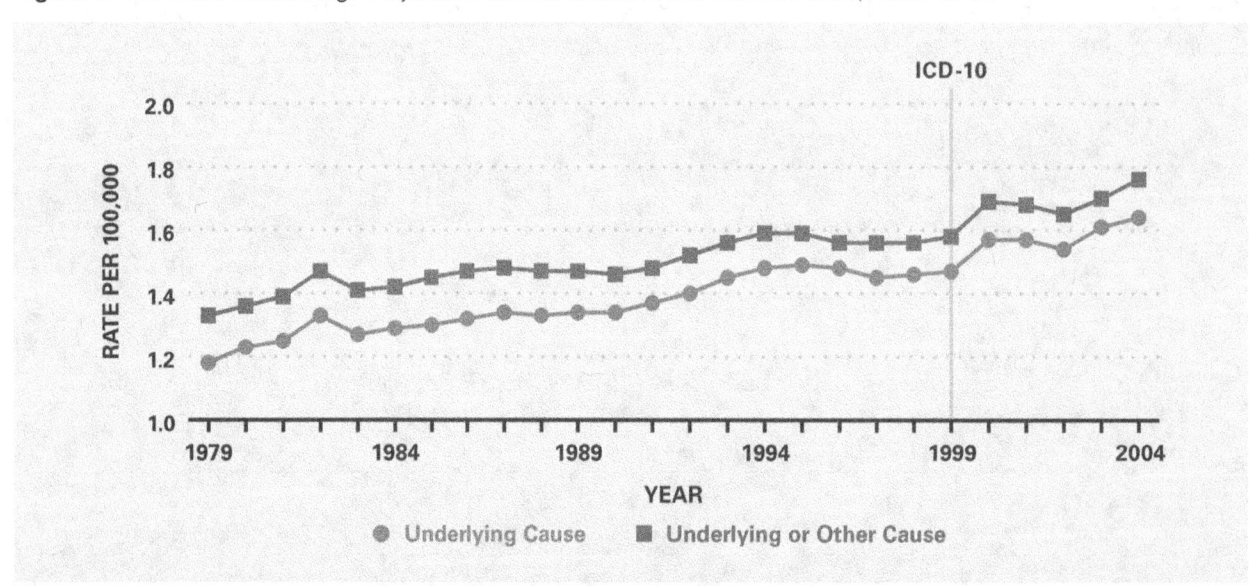

SOURCE: Vital Statistics of the United States

CHAPTER 11

Cancer of the Gallbladder

James E. Everhart, M.D., M.P.H.

About 3,000 cases of gallbladder cancer were estimated to have occurred in 2004 (Table 1). Gallbladder cancer was the only digestive system malignancy that occurred predominantly among women (nearly twice the age-adjusted rate of men) and was one of the few nongenital cancers that had a female predominance. It was predominantly a diagnosis of the elderly, with a median age of diagnosis of age 73 years, the highest of any digestive system cancer (http://seer.cancer.gov/csr/1975_2005/results_merged/topic_med_age.pdf). Age-adjusted rates were too low to draw inferences about ethnic differences in risk. Incidence of gallbladder cancer declined by 42.2 percent from 1979 to 1997, and was then stable through 2004 (Figure 1). Five-year survival increased modestly to about 9 percent. Outpatient and inpatient data were too sparse to draw inferences, except that the rate of hospitalization with gallbladder cancer declined substantially until the mid-1990s and has been stable since (Figure 2).

Because of low survival, gallbladder cancer mortality was similar to incidence. As underlying cause, there were nearly 2,000 deaths in 2004 and just under 11,000 YPLL prior to age 75 years (Table 3), which reflects the older age at which gallbladder cancer occurred. Rates were 6.8 times as high in the oldest age group (65 years and older) as among those ages 45–64 years. Age-adjusted mortality rates were higher for blacks than whites, and for females than males. The death rate for gallbladder cancer declined by 47 percent between 1979 and 2004 (Figure 3). Because gallstones are the major recognized risk factor for gallbladder cancer, it is of interest that there was a similar decline (56.1 percent) in gallstone disease-related mortality over that period.

Table 1. Gallbladder Cancer: Number of Cases and Incidence Rates by Age, Race/Ethnicity, and Sex, 2004

DEMOGRAPHIC CHARACTERISTICS		Number of Cases	INCIDENCE PER 100,000	
			Unadjusted	Age-Adjusted
AGE (Years)	Under 15	—	—	—
	15–44	79	0.1	—
	45–64	850	1.2	—
	65+	2,257	6.6	—
RACE/ETHNICITY	Non-Hispanic White	2,129	1.1	0.9
	Non-Hispanic Black	356	1.0	1.5
	Hispanic	348	0.9	1.9
	Asian/Pacific Islander	142	1.2	1.4
	American Indian/Alaska Native	—	—	—
SEX	Female	2,180	1.5	1.4
	Male	867	0.6	0.8
TOTAL		3,034	1.1	—

SOURCE: Surveillance, Epidemiology, and End Results (SEER) Program

Figure 1. Gallbladder Cancer: Age-Adjusted Incidence Rates and 5-Year Survival Rates, 1979–2004

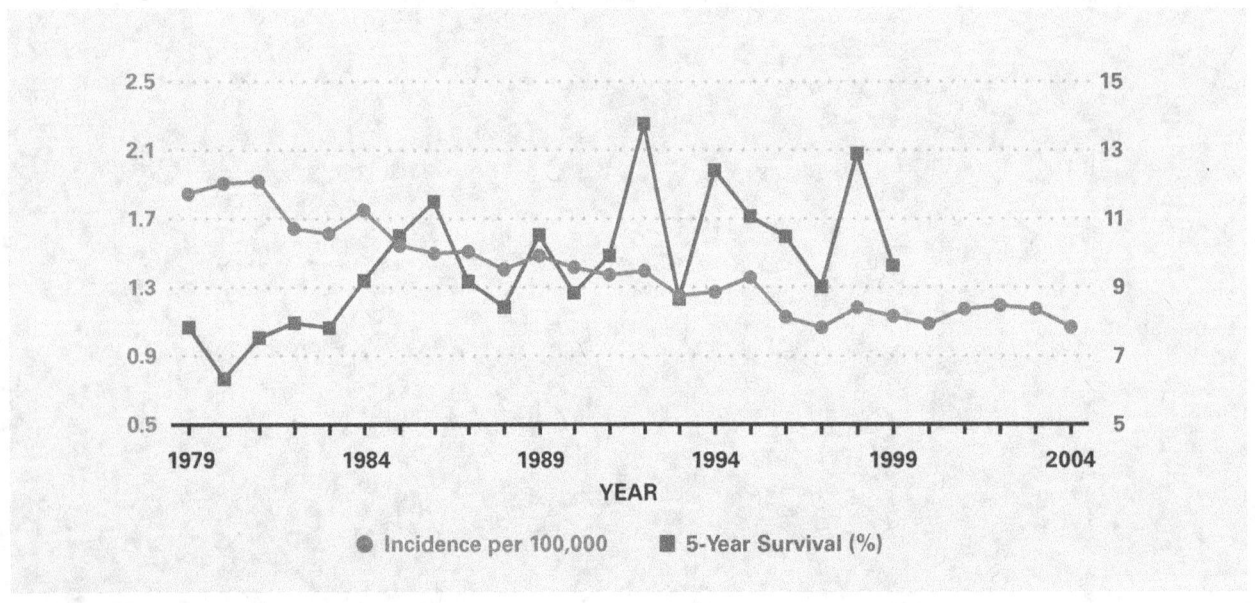

SOURCE: Surveillance, Epidemiology, and End Results (SEER) Program

Table 2. Gallbladder Cancer: Number and Age-Adjusted Rates of Ambulatory Care Visits and Hospital Discharges With First-Listed and All-Listed Diagnoses by Age, Race, and Sex in the United States, 2004

DEMOGRAPHIC CHARACTERISTICS		AMBULATORY CARE VISITS				HOSPITAL DISCHARGES			
		First-Listed Diagnosis		All-Listed Diagnoses		First-Listed Diagnosis		All-Listed Diagnoses	
		Number in Thousands	Rate per 100,000	Number in Thousands	Rate per 100,000	Number in Thousands	Rate per 100,000	Number in Thousands	Rate per 100,000
AGE (Years)	Under 15	—	—	—	—	—	—	—	—
	15–44	—	—	—	—	—	—	0	0
	45–64	—	—	—	—	1	1	1	2
	65+	—	—	—	—	2	6	4	11
RACE	White	—	—	—	—	2	1	5	2
	Black	—	—	—	—	0	1	1	2
SEX	Female	—	—	—	—	2	1	4	2
	Male	—	—	—	—	1	1	2	1
TOTAL		—	—	—	—	3	1	6	2

SOURCE: National Ambulatory Medical Care Survey (NAMCS) and National Hospital Ambulatory Medical Care Survey (NHAMCS) (3-year average, 2003–2005), and Healthcare Cost and Utilization Project Nationwide Inpatient Sample (HCUP NIS)

Figure 2. Gallbladder Cancer: Age-Adjusted Rates of Ambulatory Care Visits and Hospital Discharges With All-Listed Diagnoses in the United States, 1979–2004 (Ambulatory Care Visit Data Unavailable)

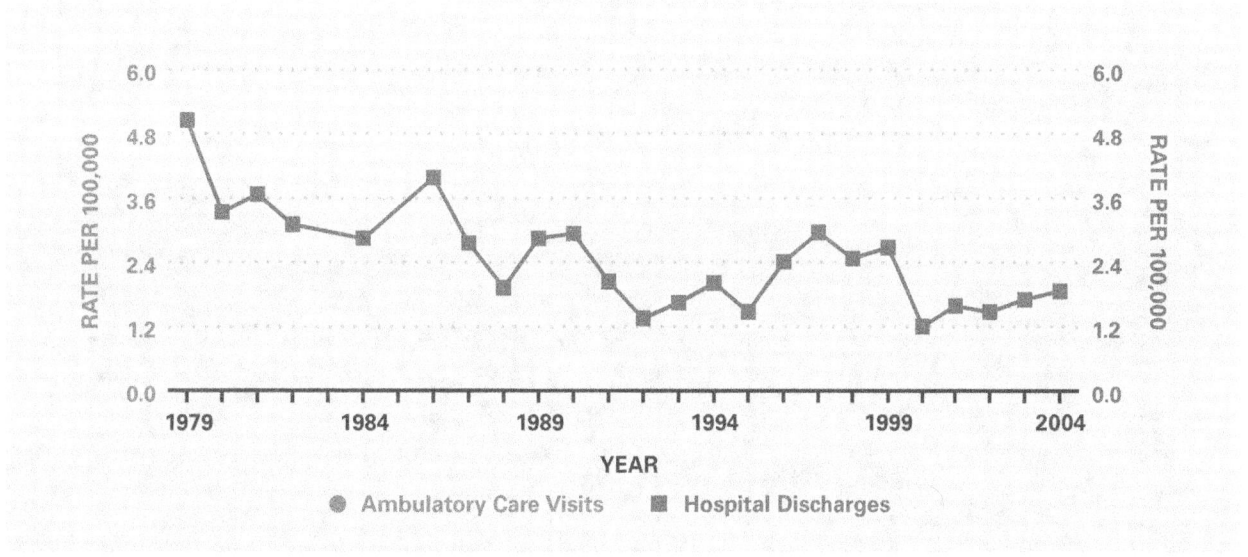

SOURCE: National Ambulatory Medical Care Survey (NAMCS) and National Hospital Ambulatory Medical Care Survey (NHAMCS) (averages 1992–1993, 1994–1996, 1997–1999, 2000–2002, 2003–2005), and National Hospital Discharge Survey (NHDS)

Table 3. Gallbladder Cancer: Number and Age-Adjusted Rates of Deaths and Years of Potential Life Lost (to Age 75) by Age, Race, and Sex in the United States, 2004

DEMOGRAPHIC CHARACTERISTICS		UNDERLYING CAUSE			UNDERLYING OR OTHER CAUSE	
		Number of Deaths	Rate per 100,000	Years of Potential Life Lost in Thousands	Number of Deaths	Rate per 100,000
AGE (Years)	Under 15	—	—	—	—	—
	15–44	41	0.0	1.5	44	0.0
	45–64	422	0.6	7.1	443	0.6
	65+	1,476	4.1	2.3	1,585	4.4
RACE	White	1,600	0.6	8.5	1,715	0.7
	Black	227	0.9	1.6	239	0.9
SEX	Female	1,343	0.8	7.4	1,422	0.8
	Male	596	0.5	3.5	650	0.5
TOTAL		1,939	0.7	10.9	2,072	0.7

SOURCE: Vital Statistics of the United States

Figure 3. Gallbladder Cancer: Age-Adjusted Rates of Death in the United States, 1979–2004

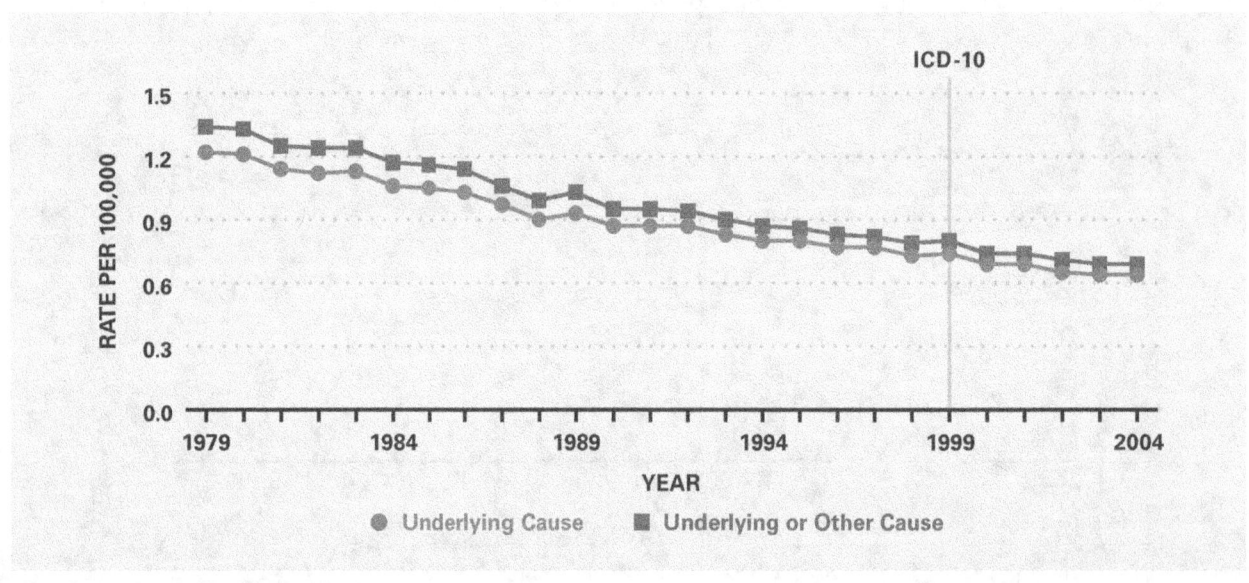

SOURCE: Vital Statistics of the United States

CHAPTER 12

Cancer of the Pancreas

James E. Everhart, M.D., M.P.H.

In 2004, 71 percent of newly diagnosed pancreatic cancers were among persons age 65 years and older (Table 1). Age at diagnosis was higher than for most other digestive system cancers, with the median being 72 years and 40 percent diagnosed at age 75 years or older (http://seer.cancer.gov/csr/1975_2005/results_merged/topic_med_age.pdf).

Incidence rates were highest among the elderly, non-Hispanic blacks, and males. Age-adjusted incidence was relatively stable from 1979 to 2004, being essentially the same in the first and last year (Figure 1). Survival from pancreatic cancer is the poorest of any major cancer, digestive system or otherwise. Nevertheless, 5-year survival increased modestly from 2 percent among persons diagnosed in 1979 to 3.8 percent among persons diagnosed in 1999.

In 2004, there were an estimated 415,000 ambulatory care visits for pancreatic cancer and 68,000 hospital discharges with a diagnosis of pancreatic cancer (Table 2). Hospitalization rates were highest among the elderly and age-adjusted rates were higher for blacks and males. While ambulatory care visits appear to have increased from 1992 through 2004, hospital discharge rates were stable from 1979 through 2004 (Figure 2).

Because of low survival, pancreatic cancer mortality was essentially the same as incidence in 2004. As underlying cause, there were 31,800 deaths in 2004 (third highest of all digestive diseases) and more than 200,000 YPLL prior to age 75 years (also third highest of all digestive diseases) (Table 3). Rates were highest in the oldest age group. Age-adjusted mortality rates were higher for blacks and for males. Death rates for pancreatic cancer remained steady between 1979 and 2004 (Figure 3).

Table 1. Pancreatic Cancer: Number of Cases and Incidence Rates by Age, Race/Ethnicity, and Sex, 2004

DEMOGRAPHIC CHARACTERISTICS		Number of Cases	INCIDENCE PER 100,000	
			Unadjusted	Age-Adjusted
AGE (Years)	Under 15	—	—	—
	15–44	878	0.7	—
	45–64	9,513	13.6	—
	65+	21,681	63.4	—
RACE/ETHNICITY	Non-Hispanic White	25,873	13.5	11.2
	Non-Hispanic Black	3,614	10.6	15.2
	Hispanic	1,929	4.8	10.4
	Asian/Pacific Islander	947	7.7	9.2
	American Indian/Alaska Native	99	5.3	8.1
SEX	Female	15,709	10.8	10.0
	Male	14,853	10.6	12.7
TOTAL		30,560	10.7	—

SOURCE: Surveillance, Epidemiology, and End Results (SEER) Program

Figure 1. Pancreatic Cancer: Age-Adjusted Incidence Rates and 5-Year Survival Rates, 1979–2004

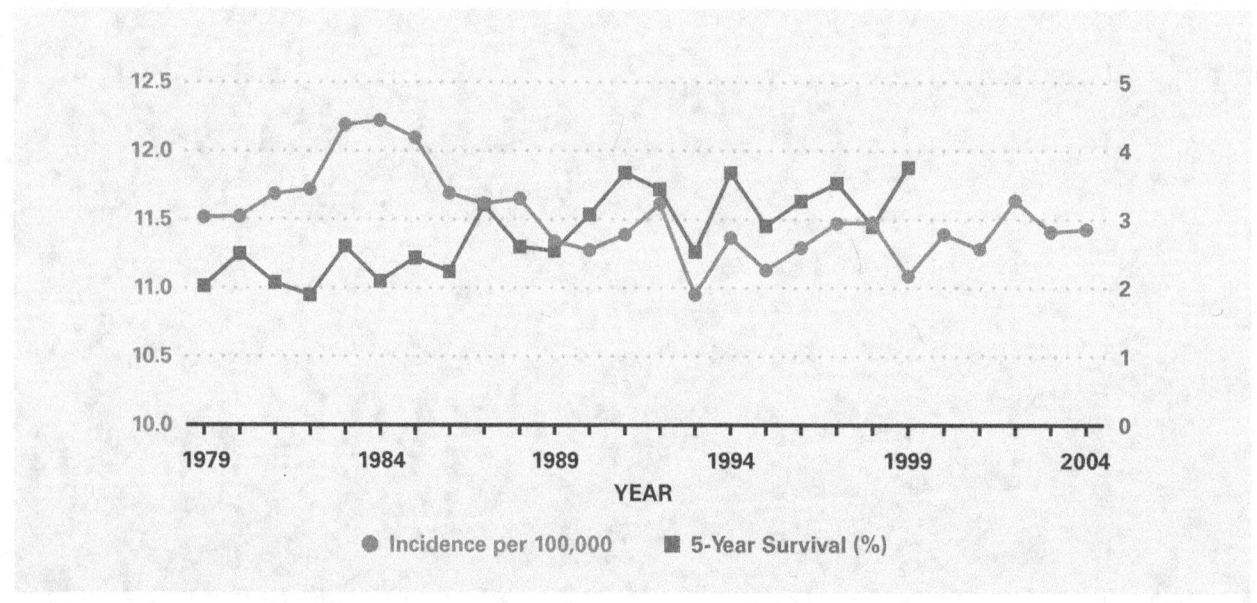

SOURCE: Surveillance, Epidemiology, and End Results (SEER) Program

Table 2. Pancreatic Cancer: Number and Age-Adjusted Rates of Ambulatory Care Visits and Hospital Discharges With First-Listed and All-Listed Diagnoses by Age, Race, and Sex in the United States, 2004

DEMOGRAPHIC CHARACTERISTICS		AMBULATORY CARE VISITS				HOSPITAL DISCHARGES			
		First-Listed Diagnosis		All-Listed Diagnoses		First-Listed Diagnosis		All-Listed Diagnoses	
		Number in Thousands	Rate per 100,000	Number in Thousands	Rate per 100,000	Number in Thousands	Rate per 100,000	Number in Thousands	Rate per 100,000
AGE (Years)	Under 15	—	—	—	—	—	—	—	—
	15–44	—	—	—	—	1	1	2	2
	45–64	154	218	162	229	12	16	23	33
	65+	230	634	251	690	21	59	43	119
RACE	White	383	148	409	158	28	11	55	21
	Black	—	—	—	—	4	15	8	30
SEX	Female	214	129	237	144	17	10	34	20
	Male	173	124	178	128	17	13	34	26
TOTAL		386	132	415	141	34	12	68	23

SOURCE: National Ambulatory Medical Care Survey (NAMCS) and National Hospital Ambulatory Medical Care Survey (NHAMCS) (3-year average, 2003–2005), and Healthcare Cost and Utilization Project Nationwide Inpatient Sample (HCUP NIS)

Figure 2. Pancreatic Cancer: Age-Adjusted Rates of Ambulatory Care Visits and Hospital Discharges With All-Listed Diagnoses in the United States, 1979–2004

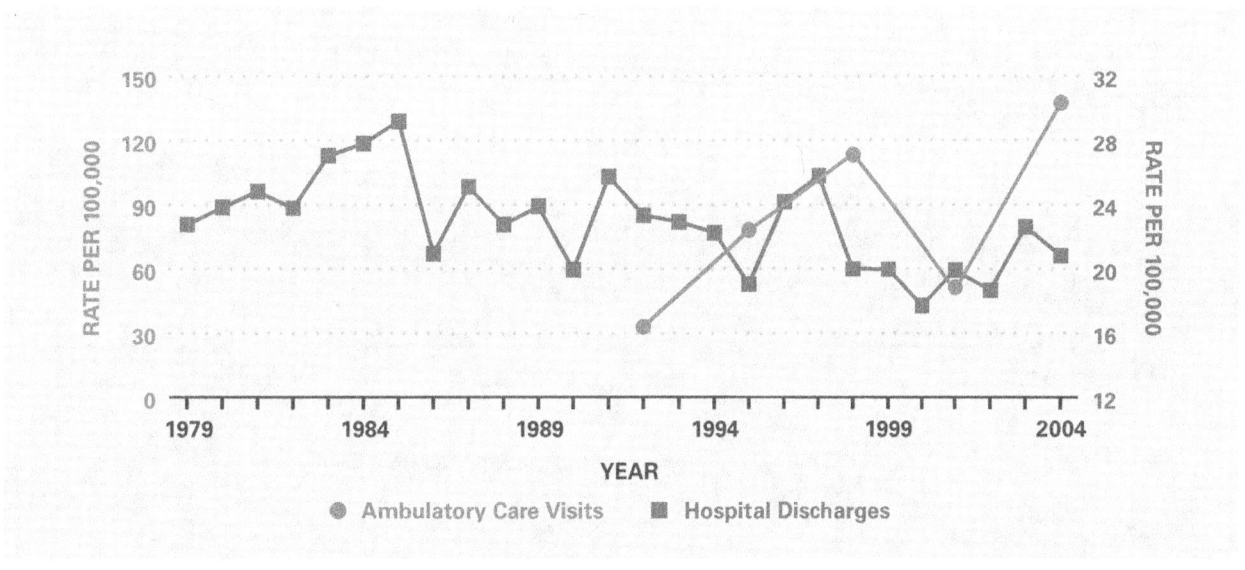

SOURCE: National Ambulatory Medical Care Survey (NAMCS) and National Hospital Ambulatory Medical Care Survey (NHAMCS) (averages 1992–1993, 1994–1996, 1997–1999, 2000–2002, 2003–2005), and National Hospital Discharge Survey (NHDS)

Table 3. Pancreatic Cancer: Number and Age-Adjusted Rates of Deaths and Years of Potential Life Lost (to Age 75) by Age, Race, and Sex in the United States, 2004

DEMOGRAPHIC CHARACTERISTICS		UNDERLYING CAUSE			UNDERLYING OR OTHER CAUSE	
		Number of Deaths	Rate per 100,000	Years of Potential Life Lost in Thousands	Number of Deaths	Rate per 100,000
AGE (Years)	Under 15	—	—	—	1	0.0
	15–44	596	0.5	20.6	606	0.5
	45–64	8,407	11.9	147.9	8,656	12.2
	65+	22,796	62.7	38.2	23,825	65.6
RACE	White	27,247	10.5	167.8	28,323	10.9
	Black	3,681	13.7	31.9	3,848	14.3
SEX	Female	16,004	9.2	83.3	16,602	9.6
	Male	15,796	12.4	123.5	16,487	12.9
TOTAL		31,800	10.8	206.8	33,089	11.3

SOURCE: Vital Statistics of the United States

Figure 3. Pancreatic Cancer: Age-Adjusted Rates of Death in the United States, 1979–2004

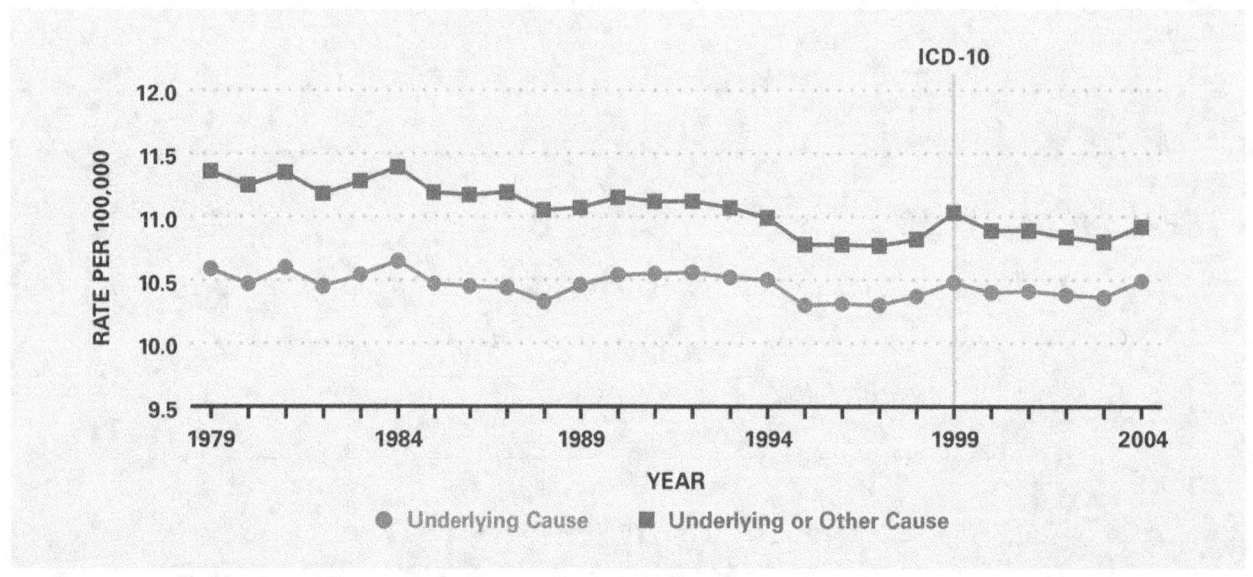

SOURCE: Vital Statistics of the United States

CHAPTER 13

Hemorrhoids

James E. Everhart, M.D., M.P.H.

Hemorrhoids are classified as diseases of the circulatory system by ICD-9 and ICD-10 (Appendix 1), but are much more often diagnosed and treated by digestive disease specialists than by those with a primary interest in the circulatory system. Therefore, burden data for hemorrhoids are presented in this report. Hemorrhoids are subclassified by anatomical location (internal or external) and whether they are complicated with bleeding, prolapse, strangulation, or ulceration. Hemorrhoids are common, and their treatment is primarily in the ambulatory care setting. In 2004, there were an estimated 2 million ambulatory care visits with hemorrhoids as first-listed diagnosis and 3.2 million visits at which hemorrhoids were an all-listed diagnoses (Table 1), which made hemorrhoids the fourth or fifth leading outpatient digestive system diagnosis (after GERD, abdominal wall hernia, and functional disorders, and essentially tied with diverticular disease). Visit rates were highest among persons age 65 years and older and among whites. Age-adjusted rates were similar for males and for females. Most hospitalizations for hemorrhoids are for surgery, which is performed most often as same-day surgery; thus, the number of hospitalizations for hemorrhoids was small relative to the number of ambulatory care visits (Table 1). As opposed to rates of ambulatory care visits, age-adjusted hospitalization rates were higher for blacks than whites. Hemorrhoids were most often listed as a secondary diagnosis (87 percent).

Age-adjusted ambulatory care visits for hemorrhoids declined slightly between the periods of 1992–1993 and 2003–2005 (Figure 1). The rate of visits in this latter period was about 20 percent lower than in the early 1980s, continuing a trend in declining outpatient visits that began in the 1960s.[1] Overnight hospitalizations with hemorrhoids listed as a diagnosis declined by about 60 percent from 1981 to 1994, and were relatively stable for the following 10 years. As a first-listed hospital diagnosis, hemorrhoids declined much more: from about 70 per 100,000 in 1979 to 13 per 100,000 in 2004.[2]

Death from hemorrhoids has always been exceedingly rare (Table 2 and Figure 2). There was a substantial decline from 1980 through 2004 in hemorrhoids noted as a diagnosis on death certificates.

Nearly 2 million prescriptions for hemorrhoids were filled at retail pharmacies in 2004, according to Verispan (Appendix 2), with topical medications such as pramoxine (pramocaine) and hydrocortisone and stool softeners such as psyllium most often prescribed (Table 3). Most persons with hemorrhoids do not seek medical care and are self-treated using nonprescription medications similar to those listed in Table 3; thus the totals in this table were a small portion of the number and cost of medications used to treat hemorrhoids.[3]

[1] Johanson JF. Hemorrhoids. In: *Everhart JE, editor. Digestive diseases in the United States: epidemiology and impact.* US Department of Health and Human Services, Public Health Service, National Institutes of Health, National Institute of Diabetes and Digestive and Kidney Diseases. Washington, DC: US Government Printing Office, 1994; NIH Publication No. 94-1447 pp. 271–298.

[2] Ibid.

[3] Ibid.

Table 1. Hemorrhoids: Number and Age-Adjusted Rates of Ambulatory Care Visits and Hospital Discharges With First-Listed and All-Listed Diagnoses by Age, Race, and Sex in the United States, 2004

DEMOGRAPHIC CHARACTERISTICS		AMBULATORY CARE VISITS				HOSPITAL DISCHARGES			
		First-Listed Diagnosis		All-Listed Diagnoses		First-Listed Diagnosis		All-Listed Diagnoses	
		Number in Thousands	Rate per 100,000	Number in Thousands	Rate per 100,000	Number in Thousands	Rate per 100,000	Number in Thousands	Rate per 100,000
AGE (Years)	Under 15	—	—	—	—	—	—	1	1
	15–44	716	569	1,131	899	8	7	57	46
	45–64	915	1,294	1,331	1,883	13	19	96	136
	65+	387	1,065	790	2,174	16	45	152	418
RACE	White	1,819	724	2,915	1,161	29	11	245	96
	Black	145	421	234	656	6	19	45	150
SEX	Female	944	621	1,745	1,132	19	12	179	110
	Male	1,092	751	1,531	1,061	19	14	127	95
TOTAL		2,036	693	3,275	1,115	38	13	306	104

SOURCE: National Ambulatory Medical Care Survey (NAMCS) and National Hospital Ambulatory Medical Care Survey (NHAMCS) (3-year average, 2003–2005), and Healthcare Cost and Utilization Project Nationwide Inpatient Sample (HCUP NIS)

Figure 1. Hemorrhoids: Age-Adjusted Rates of Ambulatory Care Visits and Hospital Discharges With All-Listed Diagnoses in the United States, 1979–2004

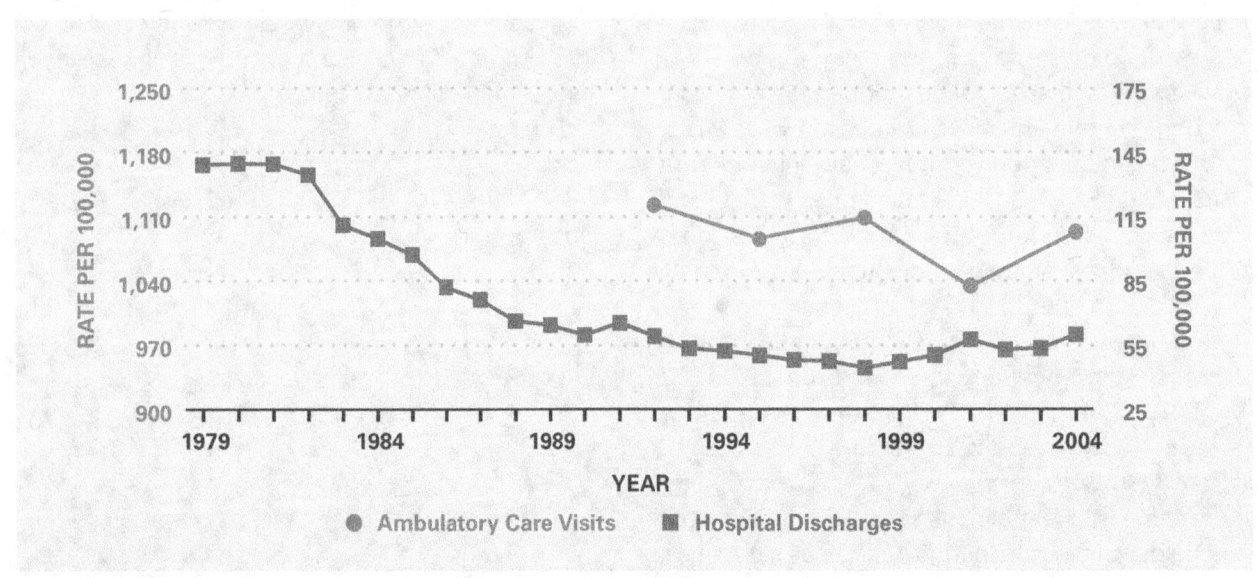

SOURCE: National Ambulatory Medical Care Survey (NAMCS) and National Hospital Ambulatory Medical Care Survey (NHAMCS) (averages 1992–1993, 1994–1996, 1997–1999, 2000–2002, 2003–2005), and National Hospital Discharge Survey (NHDS)

Table 2. Hemorrhoids: Number and Age-Adjusted Rates of Deaths and Years of Potential Life Lost (to Age 75) by Age, Race, and Sex in the United States, 2004

DEMOGRAPHIC CHARACTERISTICS		UNDERLYING CAUSE			UNDERLYING OR OTHER CAUSE	
		Number of Deaths	Rate per 100,000	Years of Potential Life Lost in Thousands	Number of Deaths	Rate per 100,000
AGE (Years)	Under 15	—	—	—	—	—
	15–44	2	0.0	0.1	5	0.0
	45–64	8	0.0	0.2	22	0.0
	65+	4	0.0	0.0	30	0.1
RACE	White	9	0.0	0.1	42	0.0
	Black	2	0.0	0.0	9	0.0
SEX	Female	3	0.0	0.0	21	0.0
	Male	11	0.0	0.2	36	0.0
TOTAL		14	0.0	0.2	57	0.0

SOURCE: Vital Statistics of the United States

Figure 2. Hemorrhoids: Age-Adjusted Rates of Death in the United States, 1979–2004

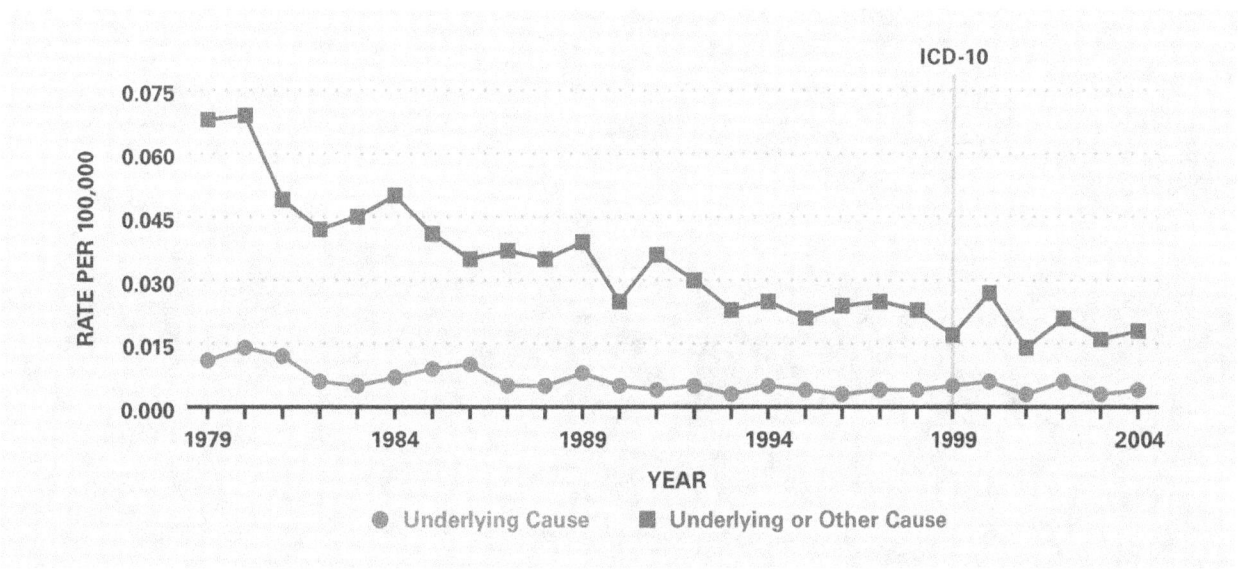

SOURCE: Vital Statistics of the United States

Table 3. Hemorrhoids: Costliest Prescriptions

DRUG	Prescription (#)	Prescription	Retail Cost	Cost
Pramoxine/Hydrocortisone	336,508	16.9%	$19,424,146	45.1%
Hydrocortisone	989,521	49.8	14,852,947	34.5
Hydrocortisone/Lidocaine	98,928	5.0	6,288,920	14.6
Docusate®	511,791	25.7	1,672,743	3.9
Hydrocodone/Acetaminophen	15,223	0.8	437,436	1.0
Oxycodone/Acetaminophen	2,550	0.1	116,818	0.3
Psyllium	7,715	0.4	80,312	0.2
Polycarbophil	14,496	0.7	43,635	0.1
Bismuth subgallate/Zinc oxide/Balsam	4,099	0.2	42,819	0.1
Ibuprofen/Hydrocodone	858	0.0	25,637	0.1
Other	4,296	0.2	39,848	0.0
TOTAL	1,985,985	100.0%	$43,025,261	100.0%

SOURCE: Verispan

CHAPTER 14

Gastroesophageal Reflux Disease

James E. Everhart, M.D., M.P.H.

In 2004, GERD was by far the most frequently first-listed digestive system condition at ambulatory care visits (Table 1), constituting 17.5 percent of all digestive system diagnoses. There were at least 6 outpatient visits with a GERD diagnosis listed per 100 persons in the United States. GERD was a common diagnosis in all age groups, although the highest rate was for those age 65 years and older. Age-adjusted ambulatory care visit rates were higher among blacks than whites and were similar for females and males. As the first-listed diagnosis, hospitalizations with GERD were not especially common relative to the frequency of outpatient visits. However, GERD was the first-listed diagnosis on only 5 percent of hospital discharges on which it was mentioned. As a result, GERD was the most common digestive system disease noted at hospital discharge and was found on 23.5 percent of hospitalizations at which a digestive system condition was listed at discharge. The pattern by race and sex of rates of hospitalization with a diagnosis of GERD were similar to the rates of ambulatory care visits. About half of all hospital diagnoses were recorded at age 65 years and older.

Rates of both all-listed ambulatory care visits and hospital discharges increased several-fold from the early 1990s to 2004 (Figure 1). Among other digestive system diseases, only viral hepatitis C saw a similar increase in medical care, but much of that increase was a result of the fact that hepatitis C was not recognized as a disease with its own ICD code until 1992. The increases in medical care for GERD began at least as early as the mid-1970s.[1] Between 1975 and 2004, the rate of all-listed ambulatory care visits for GERD increased approximately 2,000 percent. It was in the mid-1970s that better means to diagnose (flexible endoscopes) and treat (histamine-2 receptor blockers) became available, both of which stimulated recognition of the condition. Nevertheless, it is quite unlikely that all the increases in GERD-related statistics can be attributed solely to increased recognition.

Despite not being considered a fatal disease, GERD was listed as the underlying cause of more than 1,000 deaths in 2004 (Table 2), 83 percent of which occurred among persons age 65 years and older. GERD was much more often listed as a contributing cause of death, with the large majority at age 65 years and older. Mortality rates differed little by race and sex. Rates of GERD as a first-listed or contributing cause of death increased by 115 percent from 1979 to 2004, with the majority of the increase occurring during the last 9 years of that period (Figure 2).

More than 60 million prescriptions for GERD were estimated to have been filled at retail pharmacies in 2004 (Table 3), representing 48 percent of all prescriptions for digestive system disorders and more than 50 percent of their cost. The large majority of prescriptions and their cost were for proton pump inhibitors, which were the five most commonly prescribed and costliest medications. Because over-the-counter medications were not included in this tabulation, the total medication cost may have been considerably higher.

[1] Sonnenberg A. Esophageal diseases. In: Everhart JE, editor. *Digestive diseases in the United States: epidemiology and impact.* US Department of Health and Human Services, Public Health Service, National Institutes of Health, National Institute of Diabetes and Digestive and Kidney Diseases. Washington, DC: US Government Printing Office, 1994; NIH Publication No. 94-1447 pp. 299–355.

Table 1. Gastroesophageal Reflux Disease: Number and Age-Adjusted Rates of Ambulatory Care Visits and Hospital Discharges With First-Listed and All-Listed Diagnoses by Age, Race, and Sex in the United States, 2004

		AMBULATORY CARE VISITS				HOSPITAL DISCHARGES			
		First-Listed Diagnosis		All-Listed Diagnoses		First-Listed Diagnosis		All-Listed Diagnoses	
DEMOGRAPHIC CHARACTERISTICS		Number in Thousands	Rate per 100,000	Number in Thousands	Rate per 100,000	Number in Thousands	Rate per 100,000	Number in Thousands	Rate per 100,000
AGE (Years)	Under 15	693	1,139	1,504	2,473	20	33	110	182
	15–44	2,083	1,656	4,064	3,230	28	22	463	368
	45–64	2,463	3,484	6,961	9,847	53	75	1,050	1,486
	65+	1,611	4,433	5,813	15,999	58	159	1,565	4,307
RACE	White	5,567	2,267	14,964	6,002	122	49	2,513	987
	Black	1,028	2,872	2,603	8,075	21	65	342	1,107
SEX	Female	3,388	2,209	10,624	6,733	87	54	1,936	1,183
	Male	3,462	2,462	7,718	5,506	71	51	1,252	937
TOTAL		6,849	2,332	18,342	6,246	158	54	3,189	1,086

SOURCE: National Ambulatory Medical Care Survey (NAMCS) and National Hospital Ambulatory Medical Care Survey (NHAMCS) (3-year average, 2003–2005), and Healthcare Cost and Utilization Project Nationwide Inpatient Sample (HCUP NIS)

Figure 1. Gastroesophageal Reflux Disease: Age-Adjusted Rates of Ambulatory Care Visits and Hospital Discharges With All-Listed Diagnoses in the United States, 1979–2004

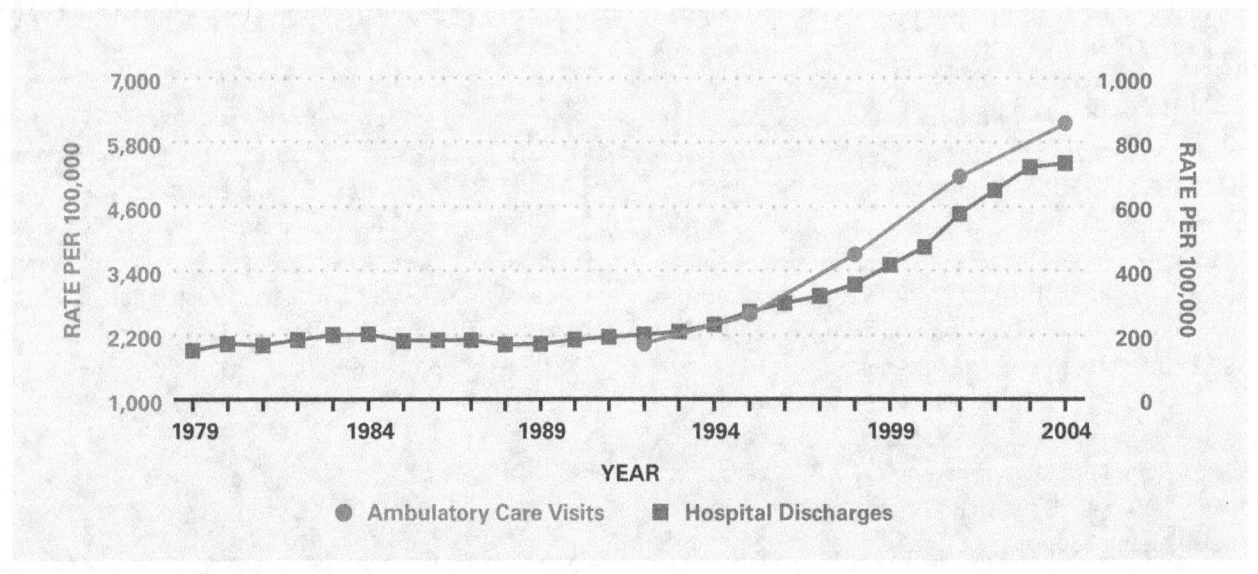

SOURCE: National Ambulatory Medical Care Survey (NAMCS) and National Hospital Ambulatory Medical Care Survey (NHAMCS) (averages 1992–1993, 1994–1996, 1997–1999, 2000–2002, 2003–2005), and National Hospital Discharge Survey (NHDS)

Table 2. Gastroesophageal Reflux Disease: Number and Age-Adjusted Rates of Deaths and Years of Potential Life Lost (to Age 75) by Age, Race, and Sex in the United States, 2004

DEMOGRAPHIC CHARACTERISTICS		UNDERLYING CAUSE			UNDERLYING OR OTHER CAUSE	
		Number of Deaths	Rate per 100,000	Years of Potential Life Lost in Thousands	Number of Deaths	Rate per 100,000
AGE (Years)	Under 15	18	0.0	1.3	106	0.2
	15–44	43	0.0	1.6	228	0.2
	45–64	135	0.2	2.5	1,034	1.5
	65+	954	2.6	0.6	6,669	18.4
RACE	White	1,033	0.4	4.7	7,273	2.7
	Black	97	0.4	1.1	649	2.5
SEX	Female	653	0.3	2.2	4,470	2.4
	Male	497	0.4	3.8	3,567	3.0
TOTAL		1,150	0.4	6.0	8,037	2.7

SOURCE: Vital Statistics of the United States

Figure 2. Gastroesophageal Reflux Disease: Age-Adjusted Rates of Death in the United States, 1979–2004

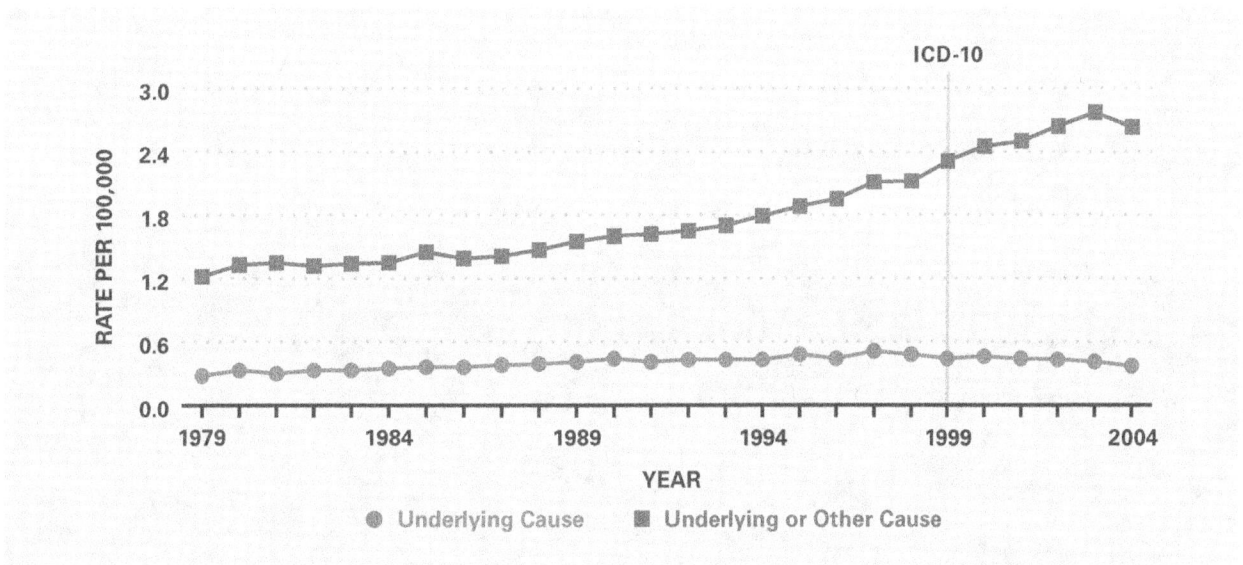

SOURCE: Vital Statistics of the United States

Table 3. Gastroesophageal Reflux Disease: Costliest Prescriptions

DRUG	Prescription (#)	Prescription	Retail Cost	Cost
Lansoprazole	14,233,183	22.0%	$2,187,235,735	28.4%
Esomeprazole	14,250,281	22.1	2,180,756,920	28.4
Pantoprazole	9,995,074	15.5	1,224,174,329	15.9
Rabeprazole	5,954,447	9.2	914,472,545	11.9
Omeprazole	6,630,268	10.3	840,514,740	10.9
Ranitidine	8,771,688	13.6	202,788,663	2.6
Famotidine	1,527,991	2.4	51,413,838	0.7
Metoclopramide	2,326,992	3.6	34,416,702	0.4
Nizatidine	187,276	0.3	26,124,573	0.3
Sucralfate	112,698	0.2	11,892,069	0.2
Other	622,786	0.8	15,976,940	0.2
TOTAL	64,612,684	100.0%	$7,689,767,054	100.0%

SOURCE: Verispan

CHAPTER 15

Peptic Ulcer Disease

James E. Everhart, M.D., M.P.H.

Peptic ulcers are coded by anatomical location (stomach, duodenum, gastrojejunum, and unspecified), chronicity, and by complication (hemorrhage or perforation). The ICD codes that cover peptic ulcers are shown in Appendix 1. In 2004, there were about 700,000 ambulatory care visits with peptic ulcer as the first-listed diagnosis and an equal number in which it was a secondary diagnosis (Table 1). Ambulatory care rates increased with increasing age, were higher for blacks than for whites, and were higher among women. When listed at hospital discharge, peptic ulcer was the first-listed diagnosis 37 percent of the time.

The frequency of outpatient and inpatient care declined for peptic ulcer disease (Figure 1), which continued a pattern that began in the 1970s, if not before.[1] Within 12 years, age-adjusted ambulatory care visit rates with a peptic ulcer diagnosis declined 68 percent, and within 25 years, hospital discharge rates declined 51 percent.

Peptic ulcer was coded as the underlying cause among 3,692 deaths in 2004 and other cause among an additional 4,604 deaths (Table 2). Nearly 80 percent of these deaths occurred among persons age 65 years and older. Age-adjusted death rates were similar for blacks and whites and were higher for males than females. Between 1979 and 2004, mortality from peptic ulcer as underlying cause declined 62.6 percent and as underlying or other cause by 68.8 percent (Figure 2). This continued at least a century of decline in peptic ulcer mortality.[2] Much of the decline in the medical significance of peptic ulcer has been attributed to the decline of *Helicobacter pylori*, which is a causative agent. This effect has likely been accelerated by the widespread adoption of acid suppressive medications (Table 3) and eradication of *H. pylori* infection by antimicrobial agents. Although antimicrobial agents are important for treatment of peptic ulcer disease, they do not appear among the most commonly used drugs, perhaps because of their short-term self-limited use. The high use of acid suppressant therapy does not differentiate indications for treatment from prophylaxis.

[1] Sonnenberg A. Peptic ulcer. In: Everhart JE, editor. *Digestive diseases in the United States: epidemiology and impact*. US Department of Health and Human Services, Public Health Service, National Institutes of Health, National Institute of Diabetes and Digestive and Kidney Diseases. Washington, DC: US Government Printing Office, 1994; NIH Publication No. 94-1447 pp. 357–408.

[2] Ibid.

Table 1. Peptic Ulcer Disease: Number and Age-Adjusted Rates of Ambulatory Care Visits and Hospital Discharges With First-Listed and All-Listed Diagnoses by Age, Race, and Sex in the United States, 2004

DEMOGRAPHIC CHARACTERISTICS		AMBULATORY CARE VISITS				HOSPITAL DISCHARGES			
		First-Listed Diagnosis		All-Listed Diagnoses		First-Listed Diagnosis		All-Listed Diagnoses	
		Number in Thousands	Rate per 100,000	Number in Thousands	Rate per 100,000	Number in Thousands	Rate per 100,000	Number in Thousands	Rate per 100,000
AGE (Years)	Under 15	—	—	—	—	1	2	2	4
	15–44	251	199	472	375	23	19	61	48
	45–64	164	233	472	668	53	75	142	201
	65+	295	812	525	1,444	104	285	283	780
RACE	White	420	171	926	371	134	52	361	141
	Black	71	251	149	491	21	70	65	218
SEX	Female	389	242	898	574	92	55	259	154
	Male	323	230	575	408	89	68	229	176
TOTAL		712	243	1,473	501	181	62	489	166

SOURCE: National Ambulatory Medical Care Survey (NAMCS) and National Hospital Ambulatory Medical Care Survey (NHAMCS) (3-year average, 2003–2005), and Healthcare Cost and Utilization Project Nationwide Inpatient Sample (HCUP NIS)

Figure 1. Peptic Ulcer Disease: Age-Adjusted Rates of Ambulatory Care Visits and Hospital Discharges With All-Listed Diagnoses in the United States, 1979–2004

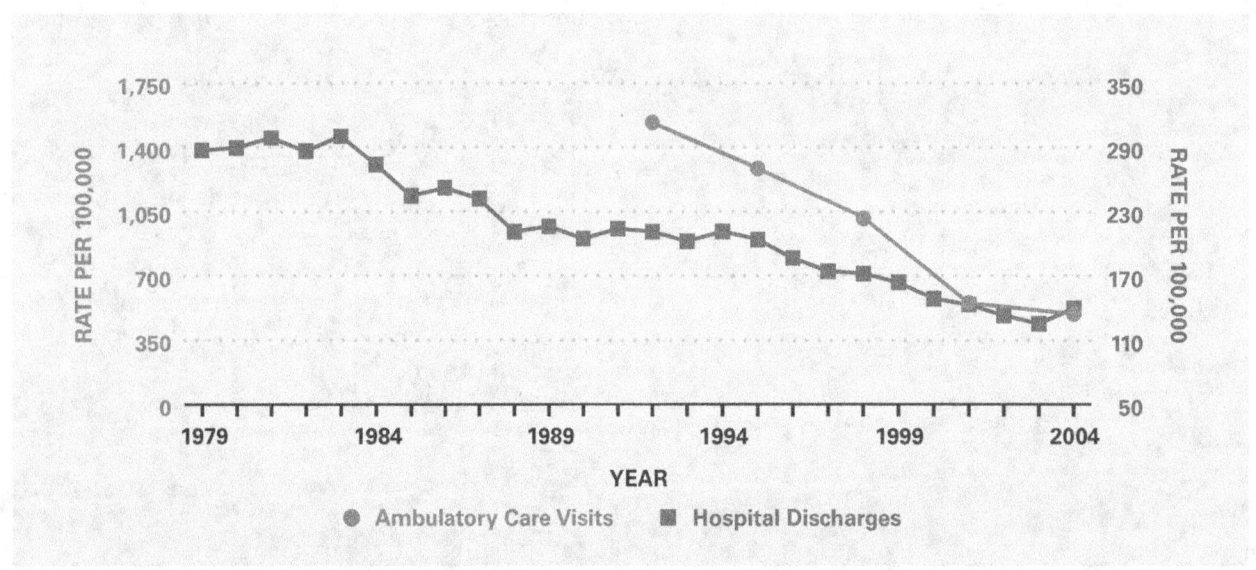

SOURCE: National Ambulatory Medical Care Survey (NAMCS) and National Hospital Ambulatory Medical Care Survey (NHAMCS) (averages 1992–1993, 1994–1996, 1997–1999, 2000–2002, 2003–2005), and National Hospital Discharge Survey (NHDS)

Table 2. Peptic Ulcer Disease: Number and Age-Adjusted Rates of Deaths and Years of Potential Life Lost (to Age 75) by Age, Race, and Sex in the United States, 2004

DEMOGRAPHIC CHARACTERISTICS		UNDERLYING CAUSE			UNDERLYING OR OTHER CAUSE	
		Number of Deaths	Rate per 100,000	Years of Potential Life Lost in Thousands	Number of Deaths	Rate per 100,000
AGE (Years)	Under 15	7	0.0	0.5	9	0.0
	15–44	118	0.1	4.3	221	0.2
	45–64	646	0.9	12.1	1,331	1.9
	65+	2,921	8.0	2.7	6,733	18.5
RACE	White	3,221	1.2	14.9	7,183	2.7
	Black	368	1.3	4.3	849	3.2
SEX	Female	1,995	1.1	7.4	4,287	2.3
	Male	1,697	1.4	12.3	4,009	3.3
TOTAL		3,692	1.3	19.7	8,296	2.8

SOURCE: Vital Statistics of the United States

Figure 2. Peptic Ulcer Disease: Age-Adjusted Rates of Death in the United States, 1979–2004

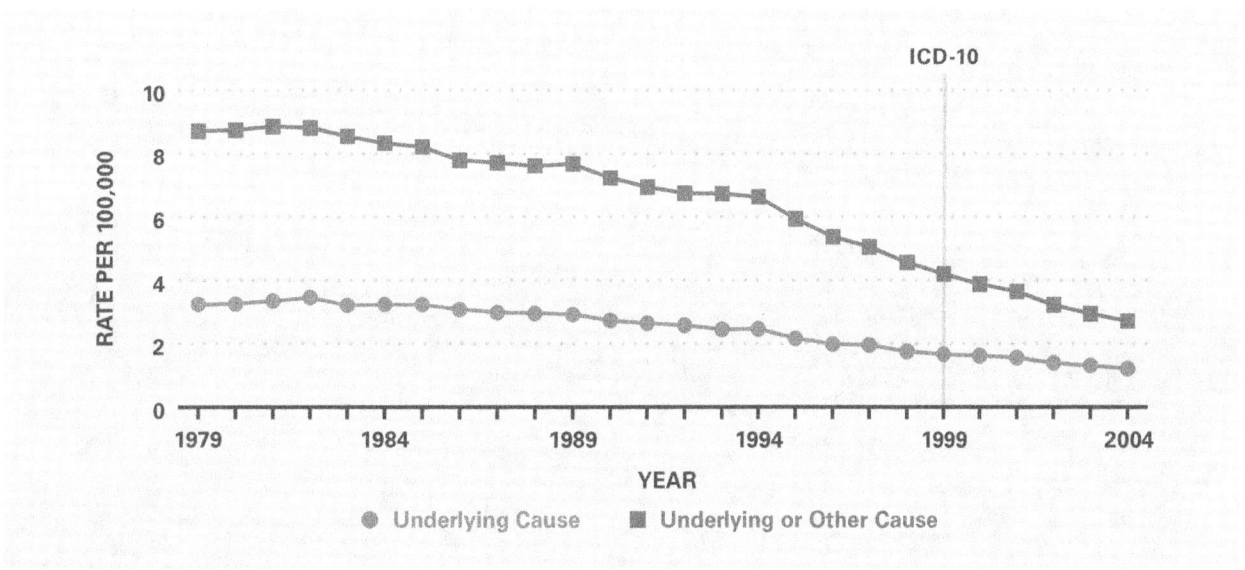

SOURCE: Vital Statistics of the United States

Table 3. Peptic Ulcer Disease: Costliest Prescriptions

DRUG	Prescription (#)	Prescription	Retail Cost	Cost
Lansoprazole	1,341,444	26.7%	$177,496,893	34.2%
Pantoprazole	1,128,002	22.5	123,697,885	23.9
Esomeprazole	680,009	13.6	85,753,825	16.5
Lansoprazole/Amoxicillin/Clarithromycin	130,482	2.6	40,749,140	7.9
Omeprazole	333,879	6.7	30,663,736	5.9
Rabeprazole	204,602	4.1	27,175,479	5.2
Ranitidine	727,492	14.5	13,039,236	2.5
Nizatidine	89,340	1.8	9,185,345	1.8
Sucralfate	157,770	3.1	5,342,588	1.0
Famotidine	135,865	2.7	3,072,170	0.6
Other	89,023	1.8	2,394,483	0.4
TOTAL	5,017,908	100.0%	$518,570,780	100.0%

SOURCE: Verispan

CHAPTER 16
Functional Intestinal Disorders
James E. Everhart, M.D., M.P.H.

Included in this chapter are separate entries on chronic constipation and irritable bowel syndrome (IBS). Other functional conditions that were either too uncommon or too nonspecific were functional diarrhea, neurogenic bowel and megacolon not elsewhere described, anal spasm, and other specified and unspecified functional intestinal disorders. These are included in the section All Functional Intestinal Disorders.

CHRONIC CONSTIPATION
In 2004, constipation was frequently noted at ambulatory care visits either as a first-listed diagnosis (3.1 million visits) or all-listed diagnoses (6.3 million visits) (Table 1), which made it the second most common ambulatory care diagnosis, after GERD. Persons under age 15 years had the highest number of visits for chronic constipation and nearly as great a rate as persons age 65 years and older. The number of ambulatory care visits for the younger age group was equal to that of intestinal infections (Chapter 2). Chronic constipation and GI infections were the two most common reasons for ambulatory care visits among children. Rates of visits with a chronic constipation diagnosis were also higher for blacks and for females. Hospitalizations with chronic constipation were uncommon, with first-listed diagnoses only 1–2 percent of ambulatory care visits. All-listed diagnoses of chronic constipation were more common—about one-tenth the rate of all-listed ambulatory care diagnoses. After many years of stable rates of medical care statistics for chronic constipation, there was a surge in both ambulatory medical care visits and hospitalizations between 1992 and 2004 (Figure 1), with more than a doubling of rates of ambulatory care diagnoses and nearly a fourfold increase in rates of hospital discharge diagnoses. The rate of ambulatory visits began to increase at least as early as 1985, when there were approximately 500 per 100,000 population.[1]

Mortality from chronic constipation is, of course, rare (Table 2). Nevertheless, in keeping with the increase in medical care, there was an increase in constipation as either underlying cause or underlying or other cause between 1989 and 2004 (Figure 2).

According to the Verispan database of retail pharmacy prescriptions (Appendix 2), in 2004, nearly half of all medications prescribed for chronic constipation were for the laxative polyethylene glycol (Table 3). Tegaserod (Zelnorm®), a medication for women with irritable bowel syndrome and constipation, was not as commonly prescribed, but was nearly as costly. Other medications were primarily stool softeners or motility agents. These data did not capture the very large number of nonprescription medications purchased for constipation.

IRRITABLE BOWEL SYNDROME
In 2004, there were 3 million ambulatory care visits with IBS noted as a diagnosis, and slightly more than half were first-listed diagnoses (Table 4). Unlike constipation, which was common among children, rates of visits with IBS increased with age only in later adulthood. Whites had more than twice the age-adjusted rate of visits as blacks. The rate of visits among females was more than 4 times that of males—the largest sex difference for any digestive disease. IBS was rarely noted as first-listed diagnosis on hospital discharge, but was much more commonly coded as a secondary diagnosis. The age, race, and sex patterns for all-listed discharge diagnosis were similar to ambulatory care diagnoses.

Age-adjusted rates of ambulatory care visits with an IBS diagnosis fell by about 20 percent between 1992–1993 and 2003–2005 (Figure 3), although the rate in the latest period was similar to rates in 1981, 1982, and 1985.[2] In contrast, rates of hospital discharges with a diagnosis of IBS fell in the mid-1980s, leveled off through the mid-1990s, and then increased by 81 percent between 1999 and 2004. IBS as underlying or contributing cause of death was exceedingly rare (Table 5), and trend data were not meaningful (Figure 4).

According to the Verispan database of retail pharmacies, in 2004, tegaserod (Zelnorm®) contributed much to the cost of IBS and was the third most widely prescribed drug (Table 6). The anticholinergic drugs hyoscyamine and dicyclomine were the most commonly prescribed drugs.

ALL FUNCTIONAL INTESTINAL DISORDERS

As a group of conditions, functional disorders were common reasons for outpatient visits, such that there were estimated to be more than 11 million ambulatory care visits noting these diagnoses in 2004 (Table 7), or about 4 visits per every 100 persons in the United States. Eighty percent of these visits were for either chronic constipation or IBS. Hospitalizations for functional disorders were uncommon, but they did commonly appear as an all-listed diagnoses. Recent increases in diagnoses with a mention of functional disorders on ambulatory care visits and hospital discharge were almost entirely due to increased rates of diagnoses of constipation (Figure 5). Chronic constipation and IBS accounted for 73.5 percent of these diagnoses. Functional disorders were coded as an underlying cause of death for 423 persons in 2004, and listed as a contributing cause for 1,766 persons (Table 8). The death rate with mention of functional intestinal conditions was stable from 1979 to 1999, when the change to ICD-10 coding resulted in a 19 percent increase that was likely a coding artifact (Figure 6).

According to the Verispan database of retail pharmacies, in 2004, there were estimated to be more than 13 million prescriptions filled at retail pharmacies at a cost of nearly three-quarters of a billion dollars (Table 9). Nearly one-third of this cost was for tegaserod (Zelnorm®). Other agents were primarily for pain, including several acid-blocking agents, or for constipation.

[1] Johanson JF. Constipation. In: Everhart JE, editor. *Digestive diseases in the United States: epidemiology and impact.* US Department of Health and Human Services, Public Health Service, National Institutes of Health, National Institute of Diabetes and Digestive and Kidney Diseases. Washington, DC: US Government Printing Office, 1994; NIH Publication No. 94-1447 pp. 567–593.

[2] Sandler RS. Irritable bowel syndrome. In: Everhart JE, editor. *Digestive diseases in the United States: epidemiology and impact.* US Department of Health and Human Services, Public Health Service, National Institutes of Health, National Institute of Diabetes and Digestive and Kidney Diseases. Washington, DC: US Government Printing Office, 1994; NIH Publication No. 94-1447 pp. 595–612.

Table 1. Chronic Constipation: Number and Age-Adjusted Rates of Ambulatory Care Visits and Hospital Discharges With First-Listed and All-Listed Diagnoses by Age, Race, and Sex in the United States, 2004

DEMOGRAPHIC CHARACTERISTICS		AMBULATORY CARE VISITS				HOSPITAL DISCHARGES			
		First-Listed Diagnosis		All-Listed Diagnoses		First-Listed Diagnosis		All-Listed Diagnoses	
		Number in Thousands	Rate per 100,000	Number in Thousands	Rate per 100,000	Number in Thousands	Rate per 100,000	Number in Thousands	Rate per 100,000
AGE (Years)	Under 15	1,175	1,933	2,127	3,497	5	8	32	53
	15–44	601	478	1,397	1,110	6	5	106	84
	45–64	492	696	1,112	1,572	8	11	164	231
	65+	880	2,423	1,671	4,599	18	50	399	1,097
RACE	White	2,582	1,064	5,057	2,100	28	11	534	209
	Black	430	1,011	990	2,620	5	15	98	322
SEX	Female	1,955	1,267	4,050	2,655	23	14	434	260
	Male	1,194	866	2,256	1,657	14	11	266	206
TOTAL		3,149	1,072	6,306	2,148	37	13	700	238

SOURCE: National Ambulatory Medical Care Survey (NAMCS) and National Hospital Ambulatory Medical Care Survey (NHAMCS) (3-year average, 2003–2005), and Healthcare Cost and Utilization Project Nationwide Inpatient Sample (HCUP NIS)

Figure 1. Chronic Constipation: Age-Adjusted Rates of Ambulatory Care Visits and Hospital Discharges With All-Listed Diagnoses in the United States, 1979–2004

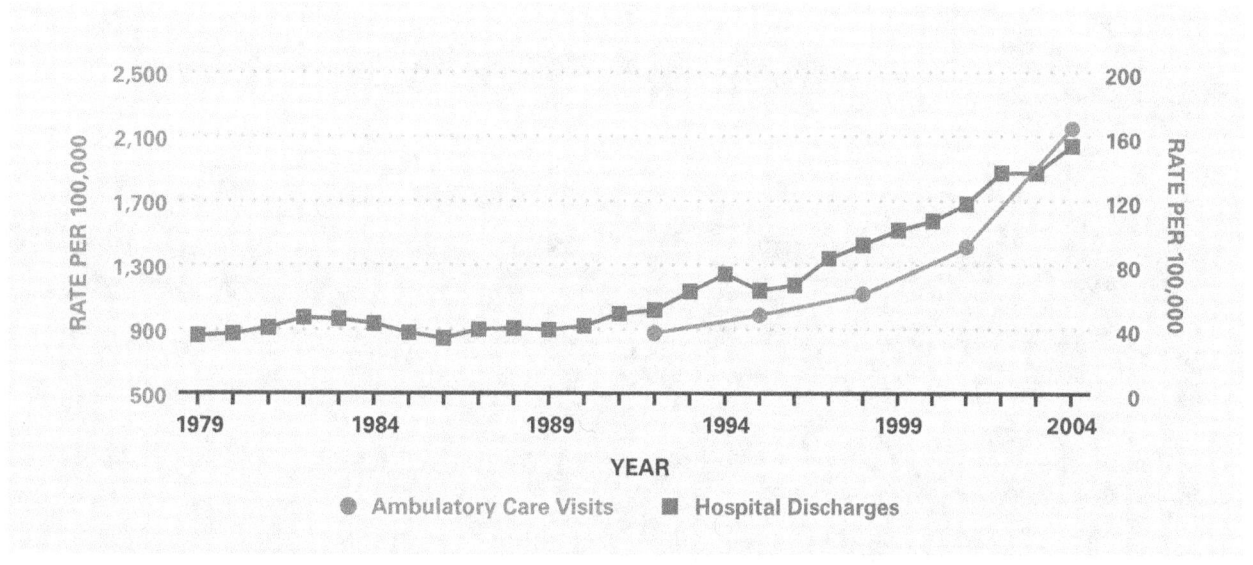

SOURCE: National Ambulatory Medical Care Survey (NAMCS) and National Hospital Ambulatory Medical Care Survey (NHAMCS) (averages 1992–1993, 1994–1996, 1997–1999, 2000–2002, 2003–2005), and National Hospital Discharge Survey (NHDS)

Table 2. Chronic Constipation: Number and Age-Adjusted Rates of Deaths and Years of Potential Life Lost (to Age 75) by Age, Race, and Sex in the United States, 2004

DEMOGRAPHIC CHARACTERISTICS		UNDERLYING CAUSE			UNDERLYING OR OTHER CAUSE	
		Number of Deaths	Rate per 100,000	Years of Potential Life Lost in Thousands	Number of Deaths	Rate per 100,000
AGE (Years)	Under 15	3	0.0	0.2	6	0.0
	15–44	11	0.0	0.5	22	0.0
	45–64	10	0.0	0.2	54	0.1
	65+	113	0.3	0.1	500	1.4
RACE	White	129	0.0	0.8	527	0.2
	Black	7	0.0	0.1	48	0.2
SEX	Female	98	0.1	0.4	381	0.2
	Male	39	0.0	0.5	201	0.2
TOTAL		137	0.0	0.9	582	0.2

SOURCE: Vital Statistics of the United States

Figure 2. Chronic Constipation: Age-Adjusted Rates of Death in the United States, 1979–2004

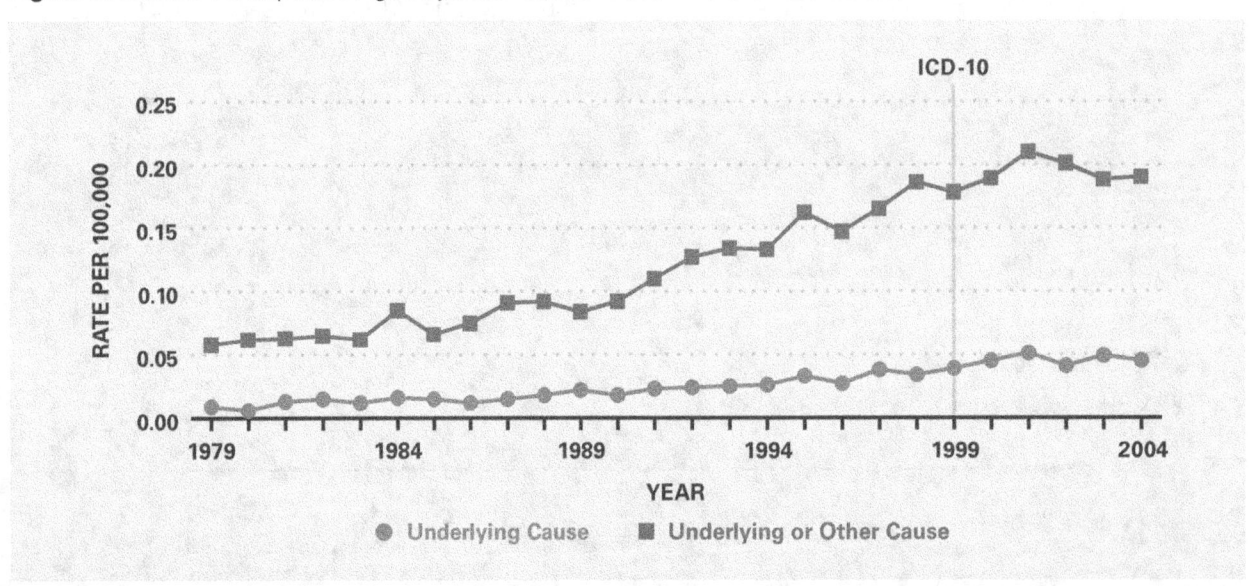

SOURCE: Vital Statistics of the United States

Table 3. Chronic Constipation: Costliest Prescriptions

DRUG	Prescription (#)	Prescription	Retail Cost	Cost
Polyethylene Glycol 3350	2,462,873	46.0%	$78,006,220	43.8%
Tegaserod	487,989	9.1	62,696,997	35.2
Lactulose	1,234,865	23.1	29,190,969	16.4
Docusate®	1,087,397	20.3	7,481,476	4.2
Methylcellulose	13,221	0.2	219,099	0.1
Magnesium Hydroxide	40,991	0.8	176,097	0.1
Psyllium	10,634	0.2	172,225	0.1
Senna®	4,085	0.1	139,618	0.1
Bisacodyl	10,271	0.2	57,569	0.0
Malt Extract	535	0.0	37,774	0.0
Other	3,432	0.0	66,635	0.0
TOTAL	5,356,293	100.0%	$178,244,679	100.0%

SOURCE: Verispan

Table 4. Irritable Bowel Syndrome: Number and Age-Adjusted Rates of Ambulatory Care Visits and Hospital Discharges With First-Listed and All-Listed Diagnoses by Age, Race, and Sex in the United States, 2004

DEMOGRAPHIC CHARACTERISTICS		AMBULATORY CARE VISITS				HOSPITAL DISCHARGES			
		First-Listed Diagnosis		All-Listed Diagnoses		First-Listed Diagnosis		All-Listed Diagnoses	
		Number in Thousands	Rate per 100,000	Number in Thousands	Rate per 100,000	Number in Thousands	Rate per 100,000	Number in Thousands	Rate per 100,000
AGE (Years)	Under 15	—	—	—	—	0	1	1	2
	15–44	724	575	1,169	929	8	6	61	48
	45–64	363	514	979	1,384	5	7	73	103
	65+	469	1,290	792	2,179	4	11	77	213
RACE	White	1,459	593	2,803	1,138	15	6	180	72
	Black	—	—	212	534	1	4	12	36
SEX	Female	1,322	867	2,531	1,649	14	9	177	112
	Male	283	201	523	373	4	2	35	26
TOTAL		1,605	547	3,054	1,040	18	6	212	72

SOURCE: National Ambulatory Medical Care Survey (NAMCS) and National Hospital Ambulatory Medical Care Survey (NHAMCS) (3-year average, 2003–2005), and Healthcare Cost and Utilization Project Nationwide Inpatient Sample (HCUP NIS)

Figure 3. Irritable Bowel Syndrome: Age-Adjusted Rates of Ambulatory Care Visits and Hospital Discharges With All-Listed Diagnoses in the United States, 1979–2004

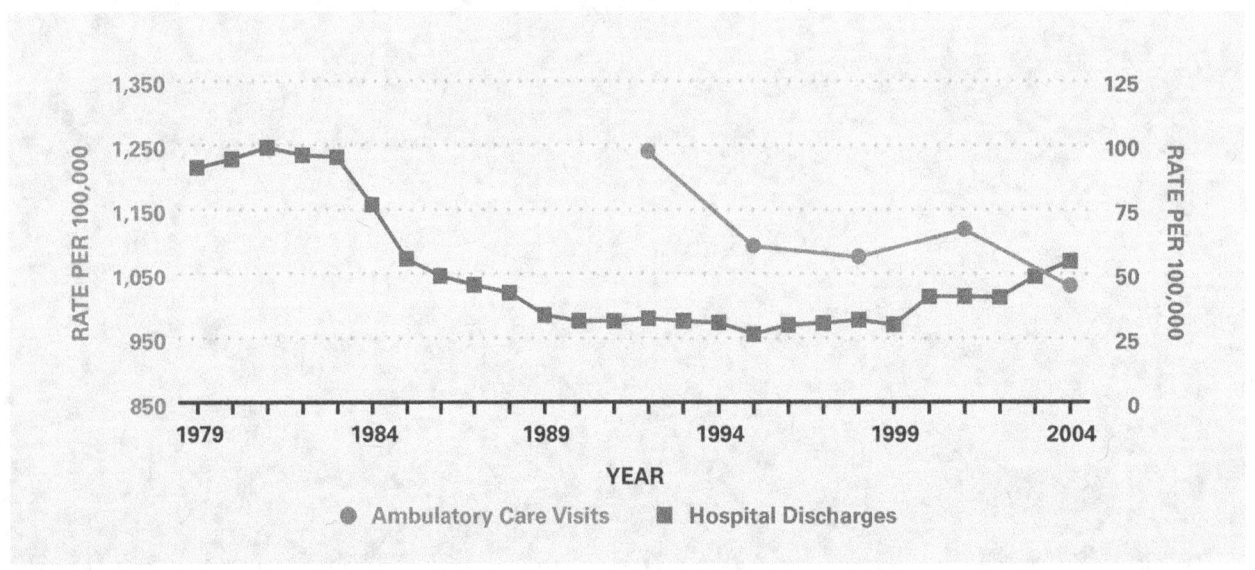

SOURCE: National Ambulatory Medical Care Survey (NAMCS) and National Hospital Ambulatory Medical Care Survey (NHAMCS) (averages 1992–1993, 1994–1996, 1997–1999, 2000–2002, 2003–2005), and National Hospital Discharge Survey (NHDS)

Table 5. Irritable Bowel Syndrome: Number and Age-Adjusted Rates of Deaths and Years of Potential Life Lost (to Age 75) by Age, Race, and Sex in the United States, 2004

DEMOGRAPHIC CHARACTERISTICS		UNDERLYING CAUSE			UNDERLYING OR OTHER CAUSE	
		Number of Deaths	Rate per 100,000	Years of Potential Life Lost in Thousands	Number of Deaths	Rate per 100,000
AGE (Years)	Under 15	—	—	—	—	—
	15–44	—	—	—	7	0.0
	45–64	1	0.0	0.0	21	0.0
	65+	19	0.1	0.0	188	0.5
RACE	White	19	0.0	0.0	210	0.1
	Black	1	0.0	0.0	5	0.0
SEX	Female	16	0.0	0.0	164	0.1
	Male	4	0.0	0.0	52	0.0
TOTAL		20	0.0	0.0	216	0.1

SOURCE: Vital Statistics of the United States

Figure 4. Irritable Bowel Syndrome: Age-Adjusted Rates of Death in the United States, 1979–2004

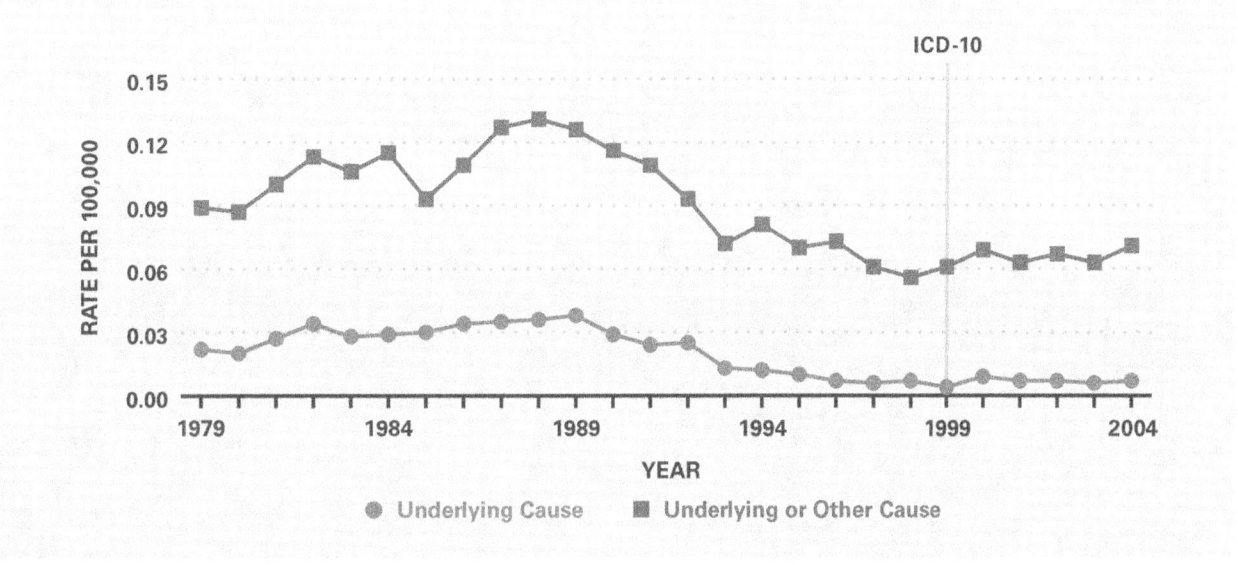

SOURCE: Vital Statistics of the United States

Table 6. Irritable Bowel Syndrome: Costliest Prescriptions

DRUG	Prescription (#)	Prescription	Retail Cost	Cost
Tegaserod	1,101,880	18.6%	$171,155,138	58.1%
Hyoscyamine	1,574,929	26.5	34,810,797	11.8
Dicyclomine	1,317,179	22.2	20,669,937	7.0
Glycopyrrolate	222,748	3.8	19,877,577	6.7
Clidinium/Chlordiazepoxide	731,965	12.3	11,525,984	3.9
Diphenoxylate	372,133	6.3	7,711,178	2.6
Pantoprazole	45,496	0.8	7,384,419	2.5
Omeprazole	76,680	1.3	5,384,300	1.8
Esomeprazole	38,526	0.6	4,546,806	1.5
Methscopolamine	70,911	1.2	4,393,505	1.5
Other	383,137	6.3	7,201,054	2.4
TOTAL	5,935,584	100.0%	$294,660,695	100.0%

SOURCE: Verispan

Table 7. All Functional Intestinal Disorders: Number and Age-Adjusted Rates of Ambulatory Care Visits and Hospital Discharges With First-Listed and All-Listed Diagnoses by Age, Race, and Sex in the United States, 2004

DEMOGRAPHIC CHARACTERISTICS		AMBULATORY CARE VISITS				HOSPITAL DISCHARGES			
		First-Listed Diagnosis		All-Listed Diagnoses		First-Listed Diagnosis		All-Listed Diagnoses	
		Number in Thousands	Rate per 100,000	Number in Thousands	Rate per 100,000	Number in Thousands	Rate per 100,000	Number in Thousands	Rate per 100,000
AGE (Years)	Under 15	1,347	2,215	2,384	3,921	10	17	48	79
	15–44	1,710	1,359	3,256	2,588	29	23	248	197
	45–64	1,127	1,594	2,700	3,820	30	42	341	483
	65+	1,762	4,851	3,308	9,104	45	124	603	1,660
RACE	White	5,039	2,057	9,690	3,980	86	35	944	373
	Black	633	1,513	1,391	3,702	16	54	169	546
SEX	Female	3,886	2,518	7,778	5,074	76	47	808	496
	Male	2,059	1,484	3,871	2,815	39	29	432	328
TOTAL		5,945	2,025	11,648	3,967	115	39	1,241	423

SOURCE: National Ambulatory Medical Care Survey (NAMCS) and National Hospital Ambulatory Medical Care Survey (NHAMCS) (3-year average, 2003–2005), and Healthcare Cost and Utilization Project Nationwide Inpatient Sample (HCUP NIS)

Figure 5. All Functional Intestinal Disorders: Age-Adjusted Rates of Ambulatory Care Visits and Hospital Discharges With All-Listed Diagnoses in the United States, 1979–2004

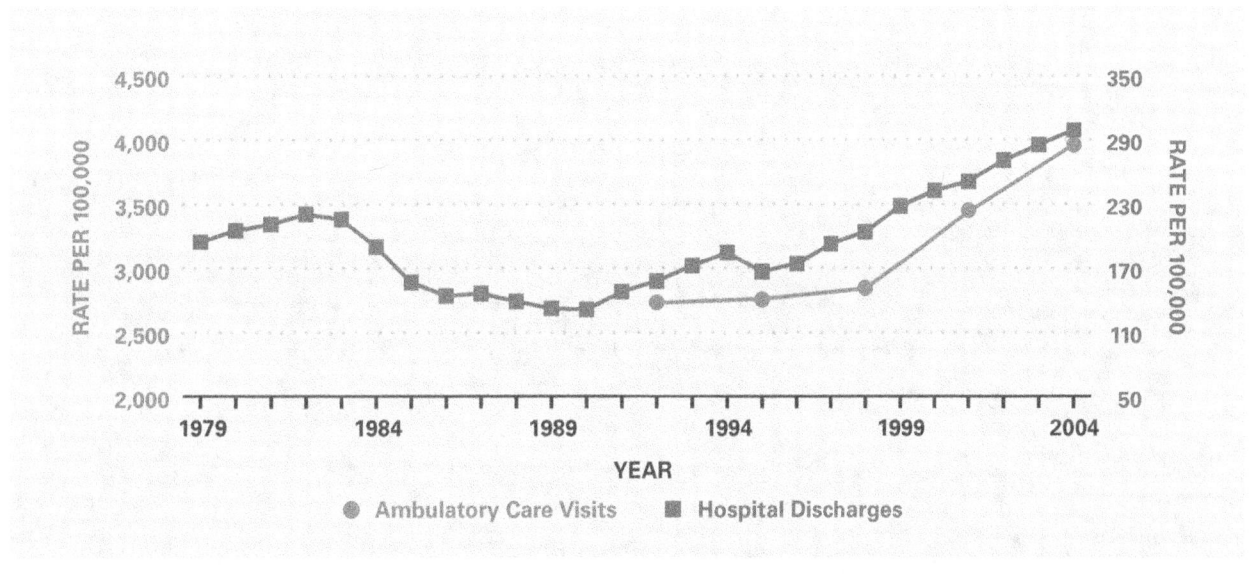

SOURCE: National Ambulatory Medical Care Survey (NAMCS) and National Hospital Ambulatory Medical Care Survey (NHAMCS) (averages 1992–1993, 1994–1996, 1997–1999, 2000–2002, 2003–2005), and National Hospital Discharge Survey (NHDS)

Table 8. All Functional Intestinal Disorders: Number and Age-Adjusted Rates of Deaths and Years of Potential Life Lost (to Age 75) by Age, Race, and Sex in the United States, 2004

DEMOGRAPHIC CHARACTERISTICS		UNDERLYING CAUSE			UNDERLYING OR OTHER CAUSE	
		Number of Deaths	Rate per 100,000	Years of Potential Life Lost in Thousands	Number of Deaths	Rate per 100,000
AGE (Years)	Under 15	6	0.0	0.4	27	0.0
	15–44	21	0.0	0.9	106	0.1
	45–64	49	0.1	0.9	335	0.5
	65+	347	1.0	0.2	1,721	4.7
RACE	White	381	0.1	1.9	1,941	0.7
	Black	36	0.1	0.5	214	0.8
SEX	Female	266	0.1	0.9	1,297	0.7
	Male	157	0.1	1.6	892	0.7
TOTAL		423	0.1	2.5	2,189	0.7

SOURCE: Vital Statistics of the United States

Figure 6. All Functional Intestinal Disorders: Age-Adjusted Rates of Death in the United States, 1979–2004

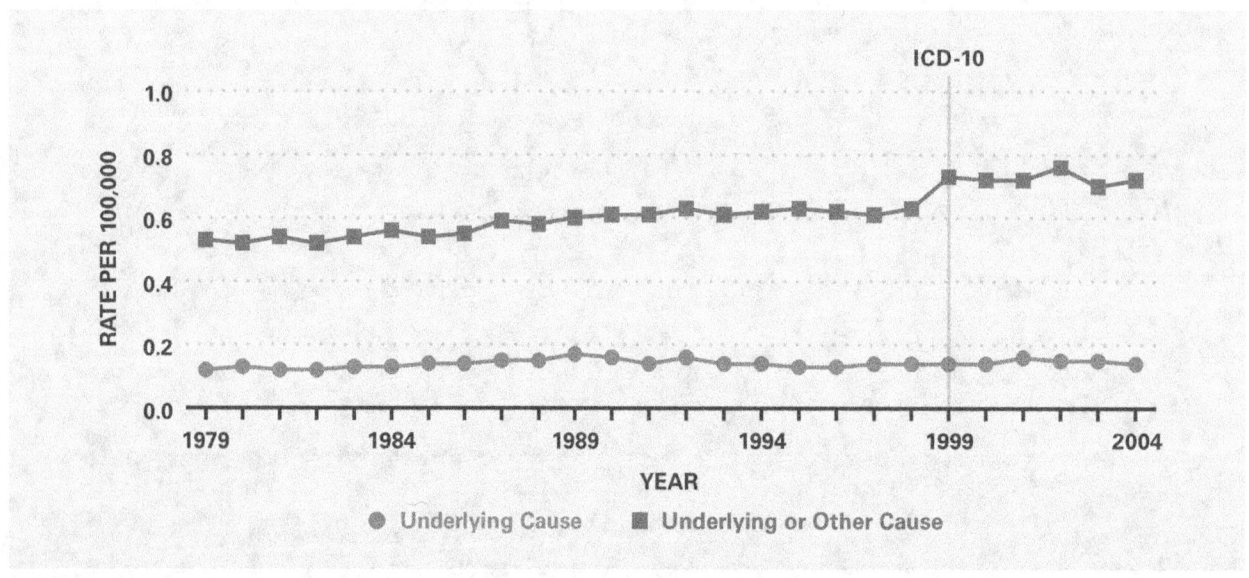

SOURCE: Vital Statistics of the United States

Table 9. All Functional Intestinal Disorders: Costliest Prescriptions

DRUG	Prescription (#)	Prescription	Retail Cost	Cost
Tegaserod	1,618,699	11.6%	$238,030,688	32.0%
Lansoprazole	695,616	5.0	85,935,464	11.6
Polyethylene glycol 3350	2,647,099	19.0	84,291,600	11.3
Esomeprazole	395,269	2.8	64,101,386	8.6
Pantoprazole	592,957	4.3	60,350,131	8.1
Hyoscyamine	1,787,325	12.8	40,443,459	5.4
Lactulose	1,278,184	9.2	30,168,691	4.1
Rabeprazole	303,450	2.2	29,843,464	4.0
Omeprazole	238,881	1.7	23,755,697	3.2
Glycopyrrolate	242,494	1.7	20,706,229	2.8
Other	4,114,833	29.6	65,854,357	8.9
TOTAL	13,914,807	100.0%	$743,481,166	100.0%

SOURCE: Verispan

CHAPTER 17

Appendicitis

James E. Everhart, M.D., M.P.H.

Being an acute surgical condition, appendicitis was not especially common at ambulatory care visits, but did account for an estimated 600,000 first-listed ambulatory care visits (Table 1), which was as frequent as those for ulcerative colitis or pancreatitis. Visit rates were nearly equal across age groups up to age 65. Rates were higher among blacks and males. Hospital discharges more accurately reflected disease occurrence. In 2004, there were an estimated 325,000 hospitalizations with a diagnosis of appendicitis, of which 91.7 percent were first-listed diagnosis. This proportion of first-listed diagnoses was higher than that of any other digestive disease and changed little over 20 years.[1] Discharge rates did not differ markedly by age. The rate among whites was twice that of blacks, while the rate for males was 20 percent greater than that for females.

Rates of ambulatory care visits increased from 1992–1993 to 2003–2005, but the more significant trends were for hospital discharges (Figure 1). Hospitalizations with a diagnosis of appendicitis declined from 1979 through 1995, continuing a decline that began at least in 1965, if not earlier.[2] Between 1995 and 2004, the trend reversed, such that there was a 34 percent increase in the rate of hospital discharges with a diagnosis of appendicitis.

Deaths from appendicitis were uncommon in 2004, with the large majority occurring at age 65 years and older, indicating a high case-fatality rate among older persons (Table 2). Mortality rates from appendicitis continued a many-year decline until 1991 (Figure 2). From 1991 onward, rates remained stable.

Because appendicitis is a surgical condition requiring hospitalization, prescriptions filled at retail pharmacies captured through the Verispan database (Appendix 2) were not frequent nor necessarily representative of the medications used in this condition. In 2004, there were an estimated 315,000 such medications prescribed, at a retail cost of $5.6 million. More than 98 percent of these medications were for pain relievers, with the rest for antimicrobial agents.

[1] Mendeloff AI, Everhart JE. Appendicitis. In: Everhart JE, editor. *Digestive diseases in the United States: epidemiology and impact.* US Department of Health and Human Services, Public Health Service, National Institutes of Health, National Institute of Diabetes and Digestive and Kidney Diseases. Washington, DC: US Government Printing Office, 1994; NIH Publication No. 94-1447 pp. 457–467.

[2] Ibid.

Table 1. Appendicitis: Number and Age-Adjusted Rates of Ambulatory Care Visits and Hospital Discharges With First-Listed and All-Listed Diagnoses by Age, Race, and Sex in the United States, 2004

		AMBULATORY CARE VISITS				HOSPITAL DISCHARGES			
		First-Listed Diagnosis		All-Listed Diagnoses		First-Listed Diagnosis		All-Listed Diagnoses	
DEMOGRAPHIC CHARACTERISTICS		Number in Thousands	Rate per 100,000	Number in Thousands	Rate per 100,000	Number in Thousands	Rate per 100,000	Number in Thousands	Rate per 100,000
AGE (Years)	Under 15	106	174	163	267	61	101	63	103
	15–44	358	284	458	364	156	124	169	134
	45–64	133	188	150	212	58	83	65	93
	65+	—	—	—	—	21	59	26	72
RACE	White	469	200	607	260	232	99	253	107
	Black	—	—	139	355	18	45	21	53
SEX	Female	260	179	372	258	126	86	144	98
	Male	341	232	410	279	164	112	172	118
TOTAL		601	205	782	266	298	101	325	111

SOURCE: National Ambulatory Medical Care Survey (NAMCS) and National Hospital Ambulatory Medical Care Survey (NHAMCS) (3-year average, 2003–2005), and Healthcare Cost and Utilization Project Nationwide Inpatient Sample (HCUP NIS)

Figure 1. Appendicitis: Age-Adjusted Rates of Ambulatory Care Visits and Hospital Discharges With All-Listed Diagnoses in the United States, 1979–2004

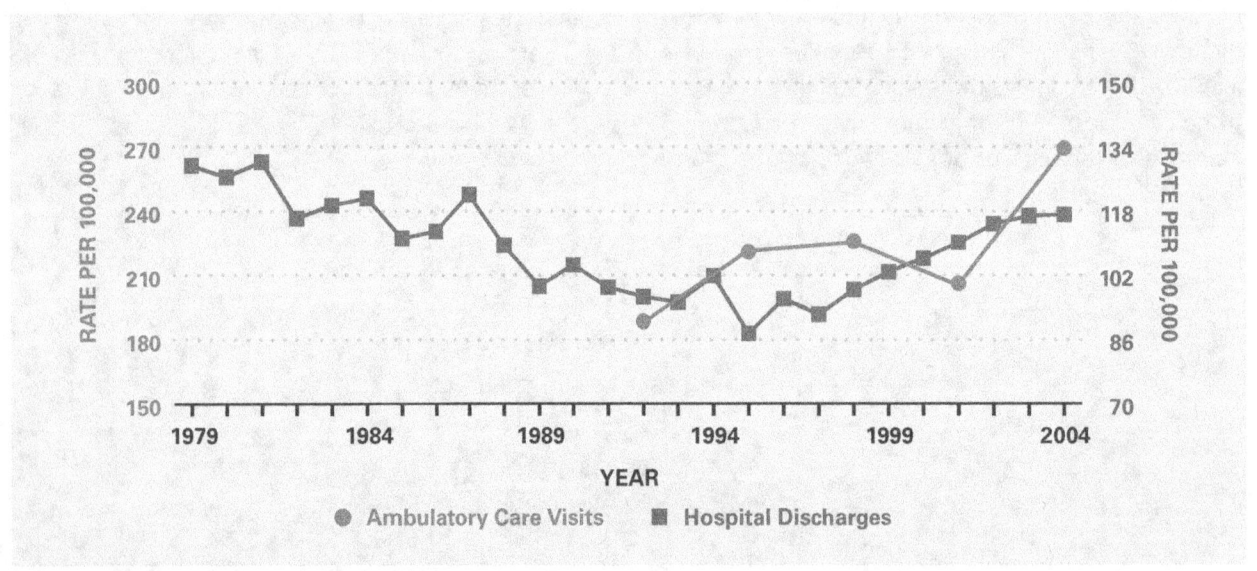

SOURCE: National Ambulatory Medical Care Survey (NAMCS) and National Hospital Ambulatory Medical Care Survey (NHAMCS) (averages 1992–1993, 1994–1996, 1997–1999, 2000–2002, 2003–2005), and National Hospital Discharge Survey (NHDS)

Table 2. Appendicitis: Number and Age-Adjusted Rates of Deaths and Years of Potential Life Lost (to Age 75) by Age, Race, and Sex in the United States, 2004

DEMOGRAPHIC CHARACTERISTICS		UNDERLYING CAUSE			UNDERLYING OR OTHER CAUSE	
		Number of Deaths	Rate per 100,000	Years of Potential Life Lost in Thousands	Number of Deaths	Rate per 100,000
AGE (Years)	Under 15	21	0.0	1.4	33	0.1
	15–44	31	0.0	1.4	45	0.0
	45–64	97	0.1	1.9	168	0.2
	65+	304	0.8	0.3	516	1.4
RACE	White	378	0.1	3.7	646	0.2
	Black	59	0.2	1.0	90	0.3
SEX	Female	200	0.1	1.4	341	0.2
	Male	253	0.2	3.6	421	0.3
TOTAL		453	0.2	5.0	762	0.3

SOURCE: Vital Statistics of the United States

Figure 2. Appendicitis: Age-Adjusted Rates of Death in the United States, 1979–2004

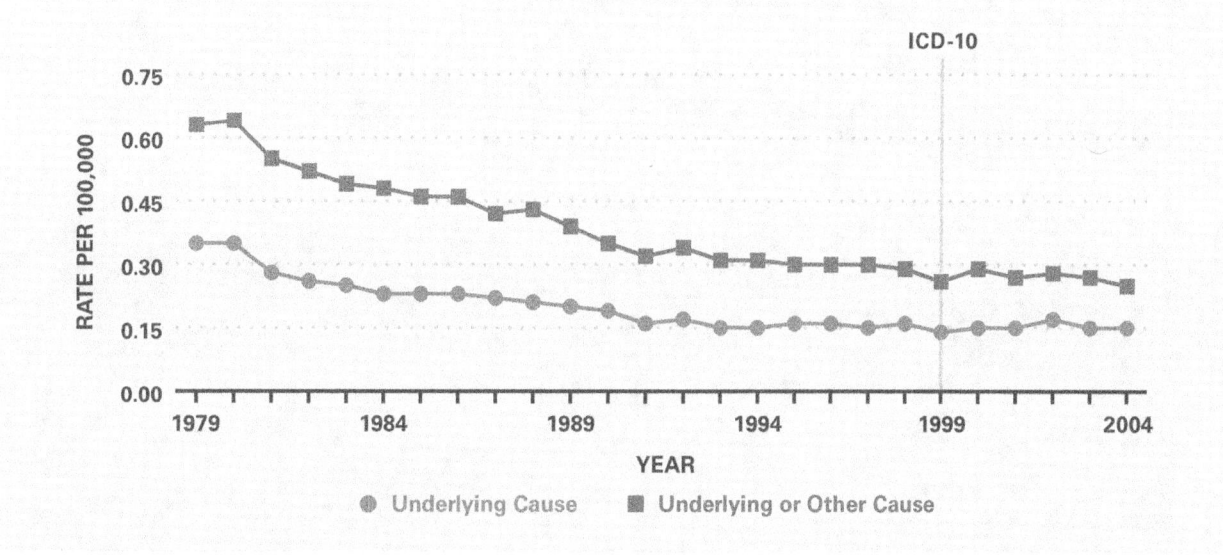

SOURCE: Vital Statistics of the United States

CHAPTER 18

Abdominal Wall Hernia

James E. Everhart, M.D., M.P.H.

Abdominal wall hernias (AWH) are coded by their anatomical location (direct and indirect inguinal, femoral, and umbilical, plus other or unspecified) and subcoded by complication (obstruction, with or without gangrene) in ICD-10. Coding was different in ICD-9, which had an odd combination of location and complication (Appendix 1). However, the individual codes match up fairly well between the two editions.

The large majority of AWH are inguinal hernias, which frequently occur as a result of incomplete closure of the inguinal canal in male infants. Hence, there was a substantial number of ambulatory care visits among children and more than twice the rate among males as females in 2004 (Table 1). However, among adults, the rate of visits increased progressively with age. Whites had a higher rate than blacks. Rates have not changed appreciably since 1975.[1] AWH was the third leading cause of ambulatory care visits in 2004, after GERD and constipation. Rates of hospital discharges with AWH were higher among blacks and there was little difference by sex.

The definitive treatment of AWH is by surgical repair. Because most repairs no longer require overnight hospitalization, the rate of hospitalizations has declined substantially, largely over a 10-year period between 1983 and 1993 (Figure 1). This decline was mostly accounted for by substantial reduction in the number of direct hernia repairs among males.[2] The same decline did not occur among females, which may account for the similar discharge rates between males and females.

In 2004, more than 1,000 persons died with AWH as the underlying cause (Table 2). The large majority of deaths occurred among persons age 65 years and older. Mortality rates were similar for whites and blacks and for males and females. Mortality rates declined between 1979 and the mid-1990s for AWH as underlying cause and more substantially as underlying or other cause (Figure 2). Mortality rates were then stable through 2004.

Because AWH is primarily a surgical condition, prescriptions filled at retail pharmacies captured through the Verispan database (Appendix 2) may not have captured the extent and nature of medication use for these conditions. In 2004, there were an estimated 3.7 million retail prescriptions filled, at a cost of $59.5 million. More than 97 percent of these prescriptions were for analgesics, with the rest for antimicrobial agents.

[1] Everhart JE. Abdominal wall hernia. In: Everhart JE, editor. *Digestive diseases in the United States: epidemiology and impact.* US Department of Health and Human Services, Public Health Service, National Institutes of Health, National Institute of Diabetes and Digestive and Kidney Diseases. Washington, DC: US Government Printing Office, 1994; NIH Publication No. 94-1447 pp. 469–507.

[2] Ibid.

Table 1. Abdominal Wall Hernia: Number and Age-Adjusted Rates of Ambulatory Care Visits and Hospital Discharges With First-Listed and All-Listed Diagnoses by Age, Race, and Sex in the United States, 2004

DEMOGRAPHIC CHARACTERISTICS		AMBULATORY CARE VISITS				HOSPITAL DISCHARGES			
		First-Listed Diagnosis		All-Listed Diagnoses		First-Listed Diagnosis		All-Listed Diagnoses	
		Number in Thousands	Rate per 100,000	Number in Thousands	Rate per 100,000	Number in Thousands	Rate per 100,000	Number in Thousands	Rate per 100,000
AGE (Years)	Under 15	160	264	417	685	5	8	24	40
	15–44	1,113	885	1,278	1,016	29	23	65	52
	45–64	1,492	2,111	1,804	2,552	60	84	124	176
	65+	976	2,686	1,288	3,545	69	189	158	435
RACE	White	3,347	1,348	4,223	1,703	130	51	290	115
	Black	287	858	437	1,275	17	54	47	142
SEX	Female	1,056	681	1,526	987	86	54	194	121
	Male	2,686	1,902	3,261	2,317	75	56	177	132
TOTAL		3,742	1,274	4,787	1,630	163	55	372	127

SOURCE: National Ambulatory Medical Care Survey (NAMCS) and National Hospital Ambulatory Medical Care Survey (NHAMCS) (3-year average, 2003–2005), and Healthcare Cost and Utilization Project Nationwide Inpatient Sample (HCUP NIS)

Figure 1. Abdominal Wall Hernia: Age-Adjusted Rates of Ambulatory Care Visits and Hospital Discharges With All-Listed Diagnoses in the United States, 1979–2004

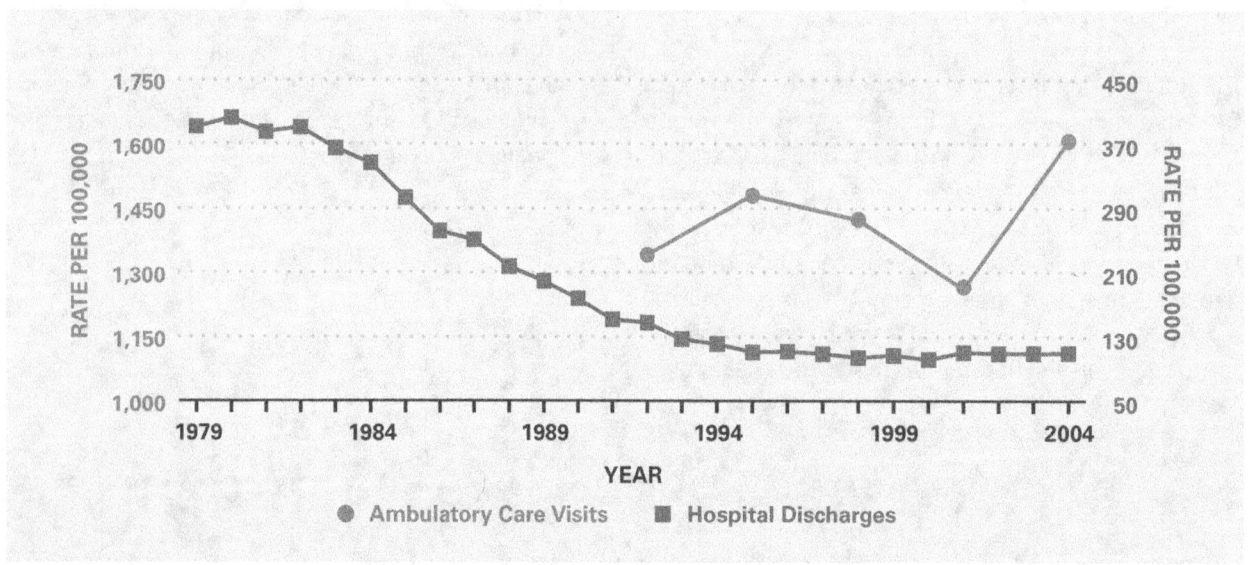

SOURCE: National Ambulatory Medical Care Survey (NAMCS) and National Hospital Ambulatory Medical Care Survey (NHAMCS) (averages 1992–1993, 1994–1996, 1997–1999, 2000–2002, 2003–2005), and National Hospital Discharge Survey (NHDS)

Table 2. Abdominal Wall Hernia: Number and Age-Adjusted Rates of Deaths and Years of Potential Life Lost (to Age 75) by Age, Race, and Sex in the United States, 2004

DEMOGRAPHIC CHARACTERISTICS		UNDERLYING CAUSE			UNDERLYING OR OTHER CAUSE	
		Number of Deaths	Rate per 100,000	Years of Potential Life Lost in Thousands	Number of Deaths	Rate per 100,000
AGE (Years)	Under 15	10	0.0	0.7	21	0.0
	15–44	43	0.0	1.6	70	0.1
	45–64	197	0.3	3.8	384	0.5
	65+	922	2.5	0.8	1,624	4.5
RACE	White	1,015	0.4	5.3	1,815	0.7
	Black	133	0.5	1.5	246	0.9
SEX	Female	670	0.4	3.2	1,132	0.6
	Male	502	0.4	3.7	967	0.8
TOTAL		1,172	0.4	6.9	2,099	0.7

SOURCE: Vital Statistics of the United States

Figure 2. Abdominal Wall Hernia: Age-Adjusted Rates of Death in the United States, 1979–2004

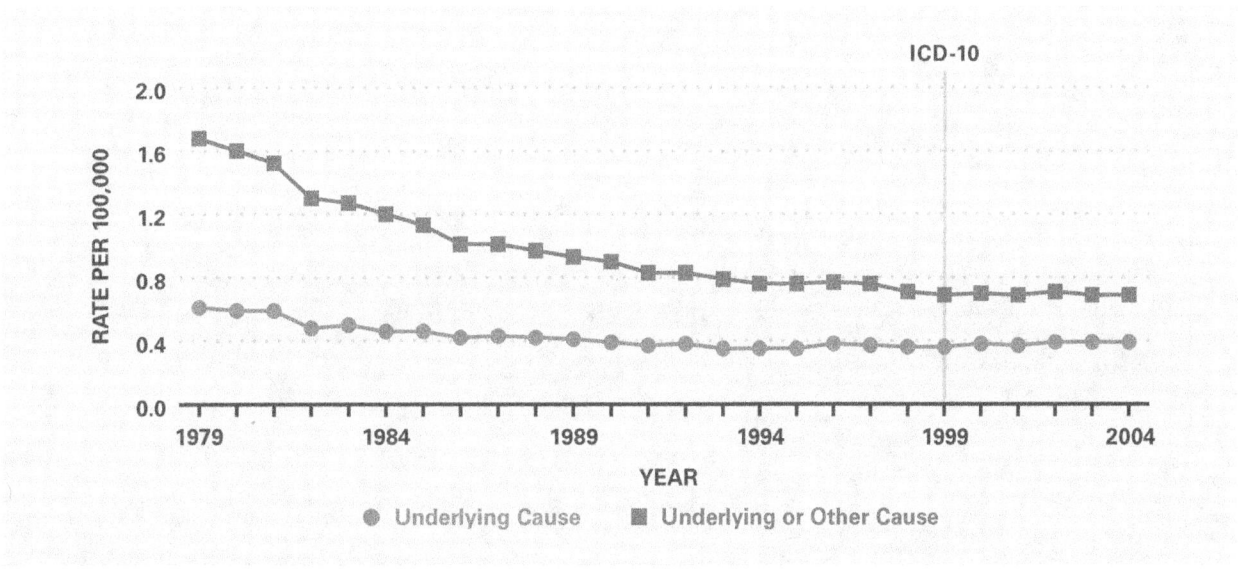

SOURCE: Vital Statistics of the United States

CHAPTER 19

Inflammatory Bowel Disease

James E. Everhart, M.D., M.P.H.

The two inflammatory bowel diseases (IBD) are Crohn's disease (also known as regional enteritis) and ulcerative colitis (UC). Adding the data for the two results in the number of ambulatory care visits, hospital discharge diagnoses, and deaths for all IBD. (Tables and figures also are shown for all IBD, but not discussed.) Most care for these chronic diseases occurs in the outpatient setting, with hospitalizations reserved for complications that might require surgery. Mortality is relatively uncommon, such that death due to GERD is more common than death due to IBD. The significant suffering from IBD is not captured well in such statistics.

CROHN'S DISEASE

In 2004, Crohn's disease resulted in more than 800,000 first-listed ambulatory care visits and more than 1 million all-listed visits (Table 1). Although Crohn's disease affects both children and older adults, more than 80 percent of visits were among young and middle-aged adults. Visits were most common among whites, and there were similar rates for males and females. Crohn's disease was the first-listed diagnosis at 57,000 hospital discharges and was mentioned as another diagnosis on nearly 100,000 other discharges. Rates increased modestly with age among adults and were higher for whites and females.

Age-adjusted rates of ambulatory care visits increased from 1992–1993 through 2003–2005 by 74 percent (Figure 1), continuing a trend that began at least as early as 1985, when the rate of office-based visits was 185 per 100,000 population.[1] Rates of hospitalization were relatively stable from 1979 through the early 1990s, but then increased modestly. Crohn's disease was uncommonly listed as the underlying cause of death in 2004, and more often as a contributing cause (Table 2). Rates increased with age and did not differ greatly by race or by sex. Between 1979 and 2004, mortality for Crohn's disease as underlying cause changed little, but as underlying or other cause increased by 53 percent (Figure 2).

According to the Verispan database of prescriptions filled at retail pharmacies (Appendix 2), mesalamine was the costliest and most frequently prescribed medication for Crohn's disease (Table 3), although not approved for this condition. Mesalamine was one of several nonspecific anti-inflammatory agents prescribed. The exception was infliximab, a monoclonal antibody for which there was a considerable cost for the modest number of prescriptions.

ULCERATIVE COLITIS

In 2004, there were about one-half million first-listed ambulatory care visits for UC and about 700,000 all-listed visits (Table 4). Visit rates were highest among young adults, and women had almost twice the rate of men. Visits were not frequent enough among other groups to provide reliable data. Hospitalizations were relatively uncommon, with 35,000 first-listed discharge diagnoses and 82,000 all-listed diagnoses.

Ambulatory care rates for UC may have increased between 1992–1993 and 2003–2005 (Figure 3), but not nearly as much as for Crohn's disease. Hospitalization rates with a discharge diagnosis of UC were relatively stable for many years, as far back as 1970, but then increased 67 percent in just 5 years, 1999–2004.[2] UC was uncommonly listed as the underlying cause of death in 2004, and more often as a contributing cause (Table 5). Mortality rates did not change between 1979 and 2004, except for a sharp drop in 1999, the year that ICD-10 was instituted for mortality coding (Figure 4).

According to the Verispan database of prescriptions filled at retail pharmacies, mesalamine and its prodrug balsalazide accounted for the majority of prescriptions and three-quarters of the prescription cost for UC (Table 6). Comparing Crohn's disease and UC, the number of prescriptions and their costs were very similar, as were the actual drugs prescribed. The major difference was that UC was treated with fewer drugs. A significant limitation of the drug data is a lack of information on infusion biologics, which have become an important and expensive treatment for IBD.

[1] Calkins BM. Inflammatory bowel disease. In: Everhart JE, editor. *Digestive diseases in the United States: epidemiology and impact.* US Department of Health and Human Services, Public Health Service, National Institutes of Health, National Institute of Diabetes and Digestive and Kidney Diseases. Washington, DC: US Government Printing Office, 1994; NIH Publication No. 94-1447 pp. 509–550.

[2] Ibid.

Table 1. Crohn's Disease: Number and Age-Adjusted Rates of Ambulatory Care Visits and Hospital Discharges With First-Listed and All-Listed Diagnoses by Age, Race, and Sex in the United States, 2004

DEMOGRAPHIC CHARACTERISTICS		AMBULATORY CARE VISITS				HOSPITAL DISCHARGES			
		First-Listed Diagnosis		All-Listed Diagnoses		First-Listed Diagnosis		All-Listed Diagnoses	
		Number in Thousands	Rate per 100,000	Number in Thousands	Rate per 100,000	Number in Thousands	Rate per 100,000	Number in Thousands	Rate per 100,000
AGE (Years)	Under 15	—	—	—	—	2	3	3	5
	15–44	405	322	505	401	33	26	64	51
	45–64	304	430	455	644	15	21	44	63
	65+	—	—	—	—	7	18	30	82
RACE	White	729	299	1,050	425	46	19	117	48
	Black	—	—	—	—	6	15	12	34
SEX	Female	462	315	665	444	32	22	84	55
	Male	385	266	512	369	24	16	57	40
TOTAL		847	288	1,176	401	57	19	141	48

SOURCE: National Ambulatory Medical Care Survey (NAMCS) and National Hospital Ambulatory Medical Care Survey (NHAMCS) (3-year average, 2003–2005), and Healthcare Cost and Utilization Project Nationwide Inpatient Sample (HCUP NIS)

Figure 1. Crohn's Disease: Age-Adjusted Rates of Ambulatory Care Visits and Hospital Discharges With All-Listed Diagnoses in the United States, 1979–2004

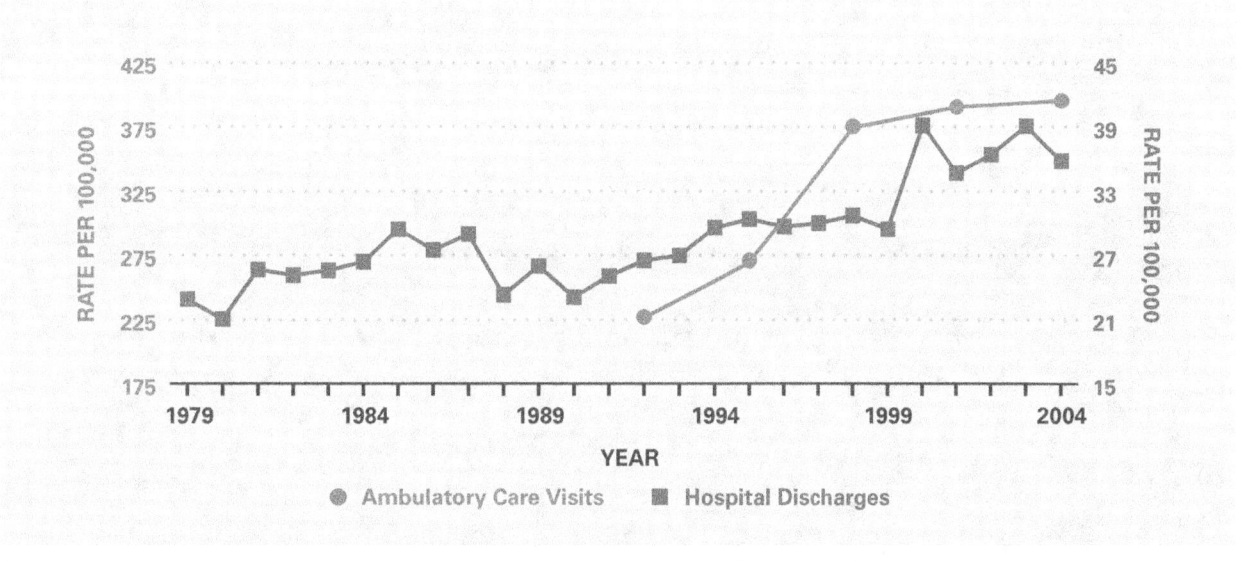

SOURCE: National Ambulatory Medical Care Survey (NAMCS) and National Hospital Ambulatory Medical Care Survey (NHAMCS) (averages 1992–1993, 1994–1996, 1997–1999, 2000–2002, 2003–2005), and National Hospital Discharge Survey (NHDS)

Table 2. Crohn's Disease: Number and Age-Adjusted Rates of Deaths and Years of Potential Life Lost (to Age 75) by Age, Race, and Sex in the United States, 2004

DEMOGRAPHIC CHARACTERISTICS		UNDERLYING CAUSE			UNDERLYING OR OTHER CAUSE	
		Number of Deaths	Rate per 100,000	Years of Potential Life Lost in Thousands	Number of Deaths	Rate per 100,000
AGE (Years)	Under 15	1	0.0	0.1	2	0.0
	15–44	70	0.1	2.8	137	0.1
	45–64	195	0.3	3.7	473	0.7
	65+	356	1.0	0.5	973	2.7
RACE	White	573	0.2	6.0	1,473	0.6
	Black	44	0.1	0.9	102	0.3
SEX	Female	371	0.2	3.5	886	0.5
	Male	251	0.2	3.6	699	0.5
TOTAL		622	0.2	7.0	1,585	0.5

SOURCE: Vital Statistics of the United States

Figure 2. Crohn's Disease: Age-Adjusted Rates of Death in the United States, 1979–2004

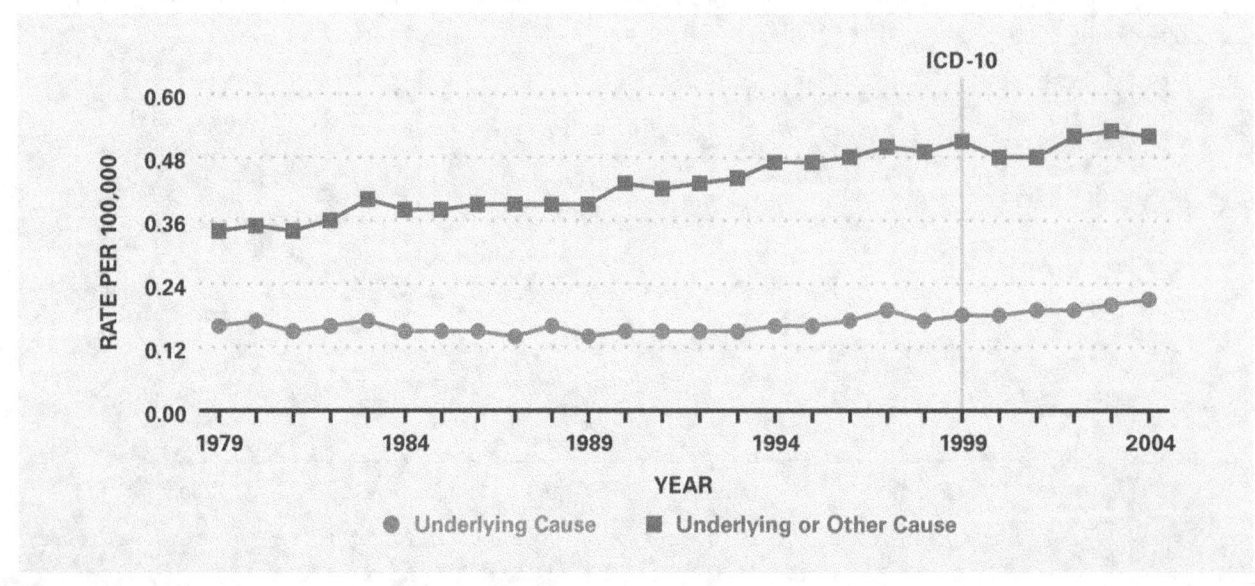

SOURCE: Vital Statistics of the United States

Table 3. Crohn's Disease: Costliest Prescriptions

DRUG	Prescription (#)	Prescription	Retail Cost	Cost
Mesalamine	701,941	37.4%	$180,555,504	69.0%
Mercaptopurine	182,978	9.7	29,004,965	11.1
Azathioprine	369,377	19.7	19,433,538	7.4
Budesonide	75,949	4.0	17,236,094	6.6
Prednisone	420,924	22.4	6,931,980	2.7
Sulfasalazine	112,215	6.0	4,230,607	1.6
Infliximab	986	0.1	2,072,089	0.8
Balsalazide	5,260	0.3	1,382,994	0.5
Methylprednisolone	6,615	0.4	337,040	0.1
Olsalazine	2,123	0.1	319,852	0.1
TOTAL	1,878,368	100.0%	$261,504,663	100.0%

SOURCE: Verispan

Table 4. Ulcerative Colitis: Number and Age-Adjusted Rates of Ambulatory Care Visits and Hospital Discharges With First-Listed and All-Listed Diagnoses by Age, Race, and Sex in the United States, 2004

		AMBULATORY CARE VISITS				HOSPITAL DISCHARGES			
		First-Listed Diagnosis		All-Listed Diagnoses		First-Listed Diagnosis		All-Listed Diagnoses	
DEMOGRAPHIC CHARACTERISTICS		Number in Thousands	Rate per 100,000	Number in Thousands	Rate per 100,000	Number in Thousands	Rate per 100,000	Number in Thousands	Rate per 100,000
AGE (Years)	Under 15	—	—	—	—	1	2	2	3
	15–44	—	—	205	163	16	13	29	23
	45–64	—	—	—	—	10	14	24	34
	65+	—	—	—	—	8	23	27	75
RACE	White	435	173	582	230	29	12	70	28
	Black	—	—	—	—	3	8	6	18
SEX	Female	306	201	483	308	19	12	45	28
	Male	—	—	232	162	16	11	37	27
TOTAL		513	175	716	244	35	12	82	28

SOURCE: National Ambulatory Medical Care Survey (NAMCS) and National Hospital Ambulatory Medical Care Survey (NHAMCS) (3-year average, 2003–2005), and Healthcare Cost and Utilization Project Nationwide Inpatient Sample (HCUP NIS)

Figure 3. Ulcerative Colitis: Age-Adjusted Rates of Ambulatory Care Visits and Hospital Discharges With All-Listed Diagnoses in the United States, 1979–2004

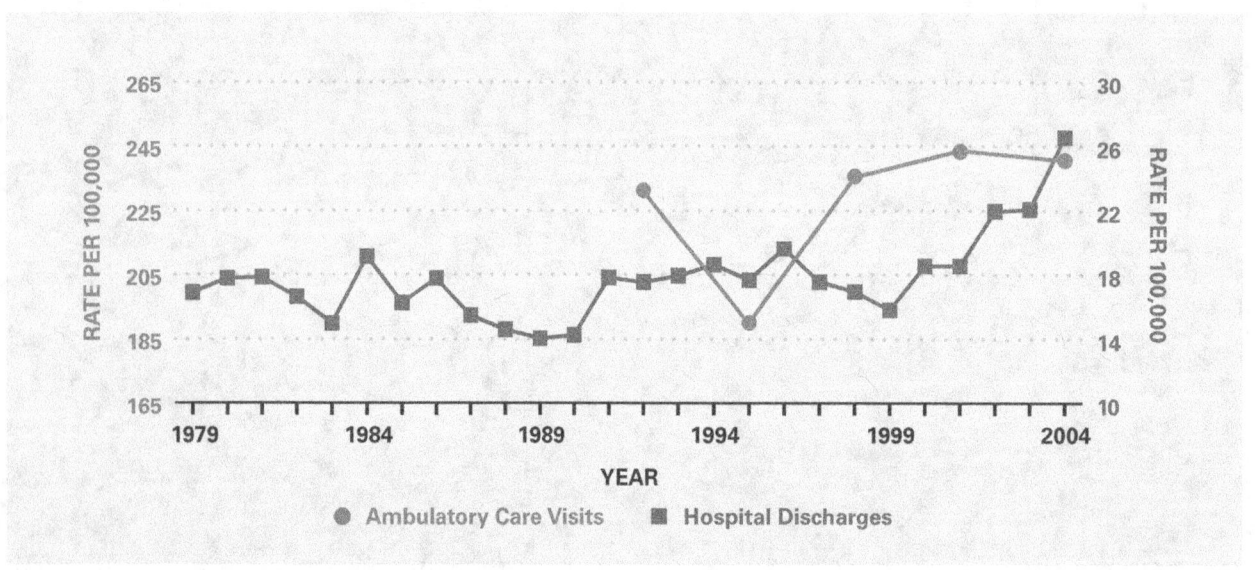

SOURCE: National Ambulatory Medical Care Survey (NAMCS) and National Hospital Ambulatory Medical Care Survey (NHAMCS) (averages 1992–1993, 1994–1996, 1997–1999, 2000–2002, 2003–2005), and National Hospital Discharge Survey (NHDS)

Table 5. Ulcerative Colitis: Number and Age-Adjusted Rates of Deaths and Years of Potential Life Lost (to Age 75) by Age, Race, and Sex in the United States, 2004

DEMOGRAPHIC CHARACTERISTICS		UNDERLYING CAUSE			UNDERLYING OR OTHER CAUSE	
		Number of Deaths	Rate per 100,000	Years of Potential Life Lost in Thousands	Number of Deaths	Rate per 100,000
AGE (Years)	Under 15	—	—	—	2	0.0
	15–44	17	0.0	0.7	65	0.1
	45–64	56	0.1	1.0	166	0.2
	65+	238	0.7	0.3	757	2.1
RACE	White	291	0.1	1.7	930	0.4
	Black	18	0.1	0.3	54	0.2
SEX	Female	168	0.1	0.9	502	0.3
	Male	143	0.1	1.1	488	0.4
TOTAL		311	0.1	2.0	990	0.3

SOURCE: Vital Statistics of the United States

Figure 4. Ulcerative Colitis: Age-Adjusted Rates of Death in the United States, 1979–2004

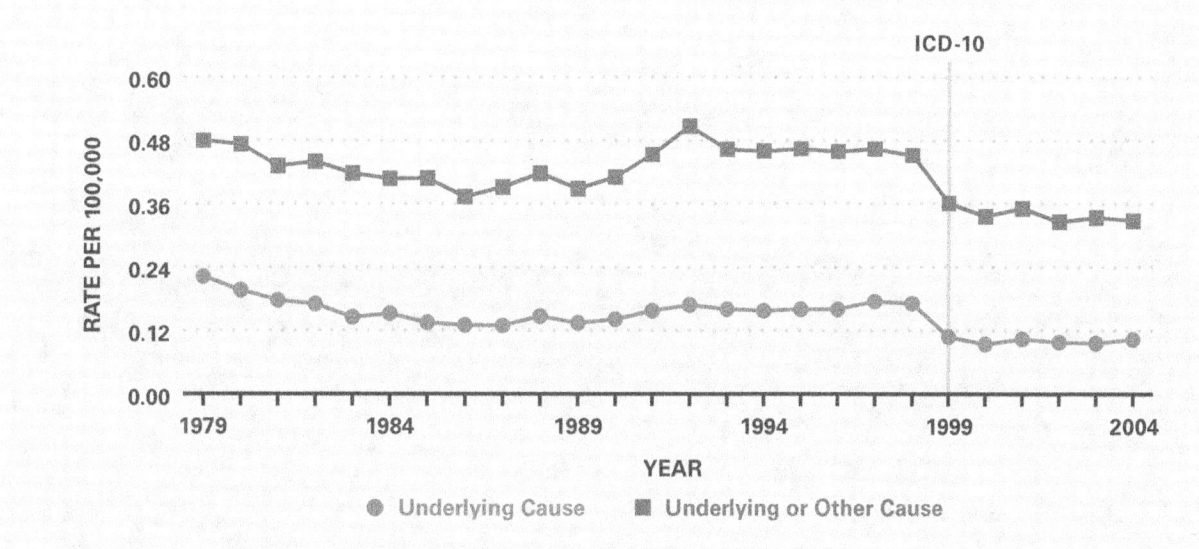

SOURCE: Vital Statistics of the United States

Table 6. Ulcerative Colitis: Costliest Prescriptions

DRUG	Prescription (#)	Prescription	Retail Cost	Cost
Mesalamine	1,080,775	49.5%	$177,226,718	65.0%
Balsalazide	213,951	9.8	57,138,781	20.9
Sulfasalazine	464,152	21.3	19,986,261	7.3
Olsalazine	57,143	2.6	9,955,396	3.6
Prednisone	350,182	16.1	4,821,998	1.8
Budesonide	15,419	0.7	3,733,906	1.4
TOTAL	2,181,622	100.0%	$272,863,060	100.0%

SOURCE: Verispan

Table 7. All Inflammatory Bowel Disease: Number and Age-Adjusted Rates of Ambulatory Care Visits and Hospital Discharges With First-Listed and All-Listed Diagnoses by Age, Race, and Sex in the United States, 2004

DEMOGRAPHIC CHARACTERISTICS		AMBULATORY CARE VISITS				HOSPITAL DISCHARGES			
		First-Listed Diagnosis		All-Listed Diagnoses		First-Listed Diagnosis		All-Listed Diagnoses	
		Number in Thousands	Rate per 100,000	Number in Thousands	Rate per 100,000	Number in Thousands	Rate per 100,000	Number in Thousands	Rate per 100,000
AGE (Years)	Under 15	—	—	—	—	3	6	5	8
	15–44	543	432	710	564	49	39	92	73
	45–64	486	688	677	958	25	35	68	96
	65+	—	—	446	1,227	15	41	56	155
RACE	White	1,163	472	1,631	654	76	31	185	75
	Black	—	—	236	764	9	23	18	51
SEX	Female	768	516	1,148	752	51	34	127	82
	Male	592	410	744	531	40	28	93	66
TOTAL		1,359	463	1,892	644	92	31	221	75

SOURCE: National Ambulatory Medical Care Survey (NAMCS) and National Hospital Ambulatory Medical Care Survey (NHAMCS) (3-year average, 2003–2005), and Healthcare Cost and Utilization Project Nationwide Inpatient Sample (HCUP NIS)

Figure 5. All Inflammatory Bowel Disease: Age-Adjusted Rates of Ambulatory Care Visits and Hospital Discharges With All-Listed Diagnoses in the United States, 1979–2004

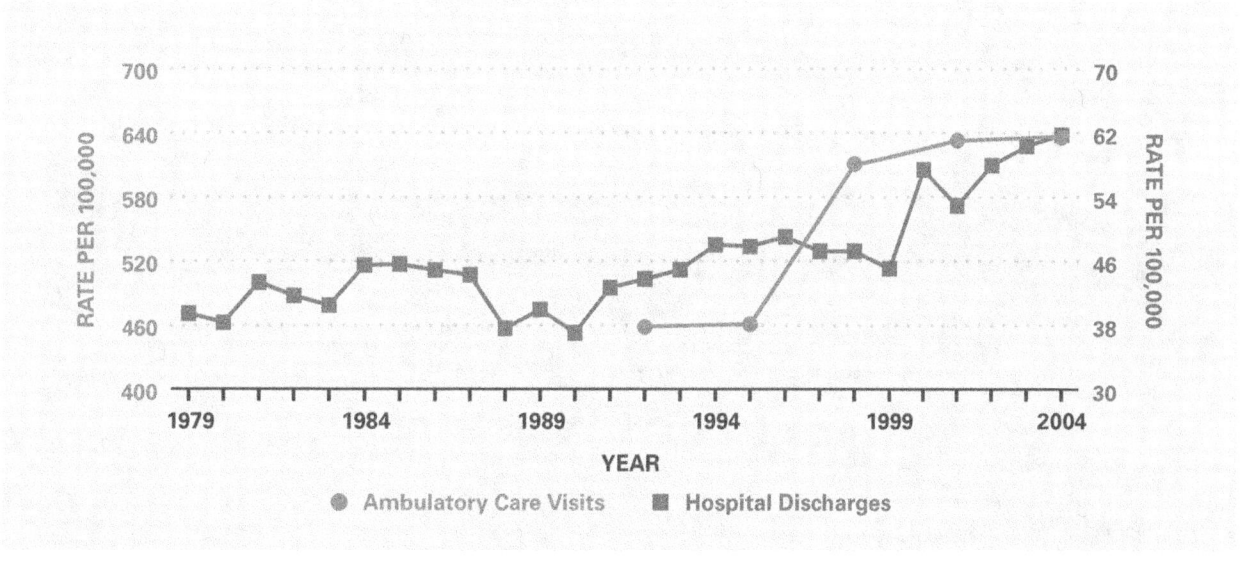

SOURCE: National Ambulatory Medical Care Survey (NAMCS) and National Hospital Ambulatory Medical Care Survey (NHAMCS) (averages 1992–1993, 1994–1996, 1997–1999, 2000–2002, 2003–2005), and National Hospital Discharge Survey (NHDS)

Table 8. All Inflammatory Bowel Disease: Number and Age-Adjusted Rates of Deaths and Years of Potential Life Lost (to Age 75) by Age, Race, and Sex in the United States, 2004

DEMOGRAPHIC CHARACTERISTICS		UNDERLYING CAUSE			UNDERLYING OR OTHER CAUSE	
		Number of Deaths	Rate per 100,000	Years of Potential Life Lost in Thousands	Number of Deaths	Rate per 100,000
AGE (Years)	Under 15	1	0.0	0.1	4	0.0
	15–44	87	0.1	3.5	202	0.2
	45–64	251	0.4	4.8	636	0.9
	65+	594	1.6	0.7	1,729	4.8
RACE	White	864	0.3	7.7	2,399	0.9
	Black	62	0.2	1.1	156	0.5
SEX	Female	539	0.3	4.3	1,386	0.8
	Male	394	0.3	4.7	1,185	0.9
TOTAL		933	0.3	9.1	2,571	0.9

SOURCE: Vital Statistics of the United States

Figure 6. All Inflammatory Bowel Disease: Age-Adjusted Rates of Death in the United States, 1979–2004

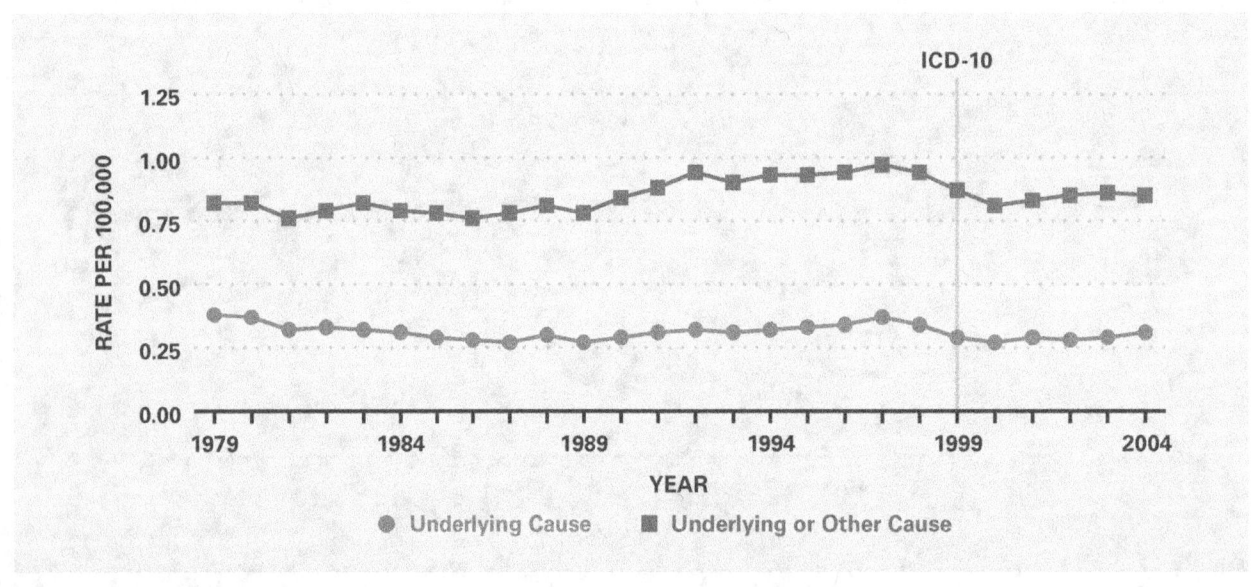

SOURCE: Vital Statistics of the United States

CHAPTER 20

Diverticular Disease

James E. Everhart, M.D., M.P.H.

Under ICD-10, diverticular disease is coded by anatomical site (small intestine, large intestine, both, or unspecified), although nearly all disease occurs in the large intestine, and by complication (perforation, abscess, or peritonitis). Under ICD-9, complications are not listed, but would presumably fall under diverticulitis, which is not a code under ICD-10.

In 2004, diverticular disease was the fifth most common reason for ambulatory care visits, after GERD, constipation, abdominal wall hernia, and hemorrhoids. Diverticular disease is generally considered a disease of the elderly, a belief that is consistent with medical care statistics (Table 1). Rates of ambulatory care visits increased with age, such that half of all visits for diverticular disease were for persons age 65 years and older. Age-adjusted rates were 18 percent higher among whites than blacks and 49 percent higher among women than men. Among digestive diseases, diverticular disease was also one of the most common reasons for hospitalization, with 313,000 first-listed and 815,000 all-listed diagnoses. Rates of hospitalization by demographic groups were similar to those of ambulatory care visits, although blacks had a higher rate than whites.

Ambulatory care visits with a diagnosis of diverticular disease increased about 18 percent between 1992–1993 and 2003–2005 (Figure 1). The rate of hospitalizations with a diagnosis of diverticular disease declined from 1982 until 1989, as it did for other digestive diseases. After several years of minimal change, rates began to increase slightly at the end of the 1990s, rising 16.4 percent between 1996 and 2004.

Diverticular disease was listed as the underlying cause of death among about 58 percent of certificates on which it was listed (Table 2). Nearly 90 percent of underlying cause of deaths occurred among persons age 65 years and older, resulting in an average of only 2.5 YPLL prior to age 75 per death. Age-adjusted death rates were modestly higher among whites and females. Mortality rates as underlying cause of death declined steadily by a total of 35 percent from 1980 through 2004 (Figure 2), which continued a decline begun in 1970 or earlier.[1]

In 2004, there were an estimated 2.8 million prescriptions at a cost of $100 million filled at retail pharmacies for diagnosis of diverticular disease (Table 3), according to the Verispan database (Appendix 2). All 10 costliest medications were for either antimicrobial agents (ciprofloxacin being the costliest and most common) or pain-relievers, led by morphine.

[1] Mendeloff AI, Everhart JE. Diverticular disease of the colon. In: Everhart JE, editor. *Digestive diseases in the United States: epidemiology and impact.* US Department of Health and Human Services, Public Health Service, National Institutes of Health, National Institute of Diabetes and Digestive and Kidney Diseases. Washington, DC: US Government Printing Office, 1994; NIH Publication No. 94-1447 pp. 551–565.

Table 1. Diverticular Disease: Number and Age-Adjusted Rates of Ambulatory Care Visits and Hospital Discharges With First-Listed and All-Listed Diagnoses by Age, Race, and Sex in the United States, 2004

DEMOGRAPHIC CHARACTERISTICS		AMBULATORY CARE VISITS				HOSPITAL DISCHARGES			
		First-Listed Diagnosis		All-Listed Diagnoses		First-Listed Diagnosis		All-Listed Diagnoses	
		Number in Thousands	Rate per 100,000	Number in Thousands	Rate per 100,000	Number in Thousands	Rate per 100,000	Number in Thousands	Rate per 100,000
AGE (Years)	Under 15	—	—	—	—	—	—	—	—
	15–44	280	222	329	261	39	31	59	47
	45–64	622	879	1,239	1,753	101	142	212	299
	65+	947	2,607	1,686	4,641	173	477	544	1,498
RACE	White	1,609	627	2,878	1,115	252	99	668	258
	Black	143	481	264	945	30	110	79	291
SEX	Female	1,284	785	2,109	1,293	181	108	493	288
	Male	580	434	1,160	865	131	99	321	251
TOTAL		1,864	635	3,269	1,113	313	107	815	278

SOURCE: National Ambulatory Medical Care Survey (NAMCS) and National Hospital Ambulatory Medical Care Survey (NHAMCS) (3-year average, 2003–2005), and Healthcare Cost and Utilization Project Nationwide Inpatient Sample (HCUP NIS)

Figure 1. Diverticular Disease: Age-Adjusted Rates of Ambulatory Care Visits and Hospital Discharges With All-Listed Diagnoses in the United States, 1979–2004

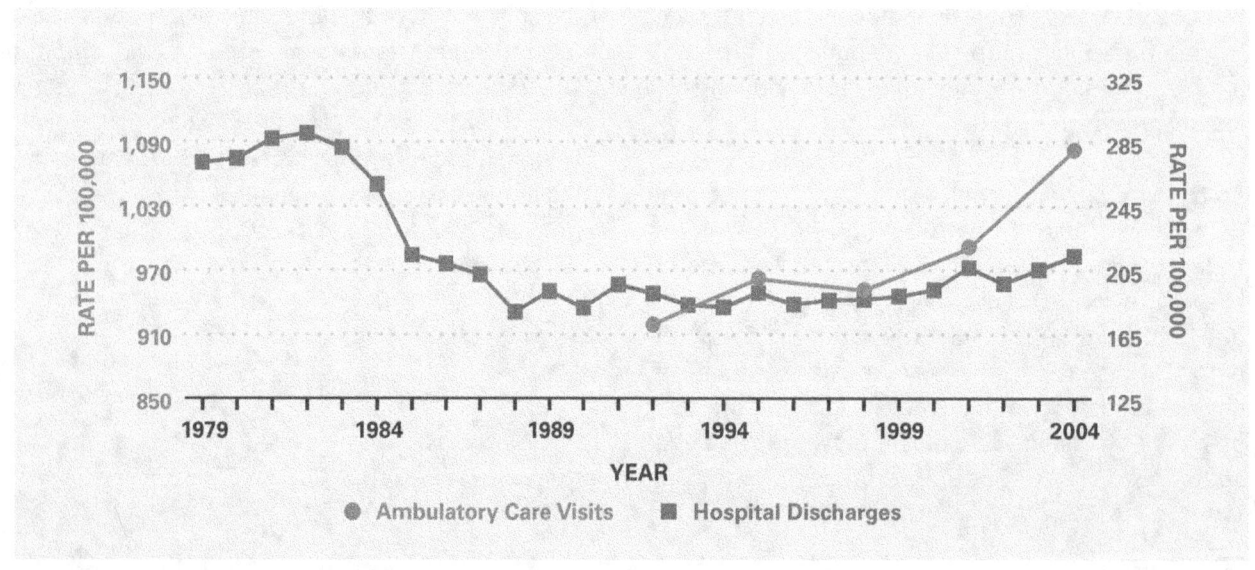

SOURCE: National Ambulatory Medical Care Survey (NAMCS) and National Hospital Ambulatory Medical Care Survey (NHAMCS) (averages 1992–1993, 1994–1996, 1997–1999, 2000–2002, 2003–2005), and National Hospital Discharge Survey (NHDS)

Table 2. Diverticular Disease: Number and Age-Adjusted Rates of Deaths and Years of Potential Life Lost (to Age 75) by Age, Race, and Sex in the United States, 2004

DEMOGRAPHIC CHARACTERISTICS		UNDERLYING CAUSE			UNDERLYING OR OTHER CAUSE	
		Number of Deaths	Rate per 100,000	Years of Potential Life Lost in Thousands	Number of Deaths	Rate per 100,000
AGE (Years)	Under 15	—	—	—	—	—
	15–44	39	0.0	1.4	58	0.0
	45–64	306	0.4	5.1	505	0.7
	65+	3,027	8.3	2.1	5,238	14.4
RACE	White	3,084	1.2	7.2	5,308	2.0
	Black	243	1.0	1.1	410	1.7
SEX	Female	2,299	1.2	4.2	3,867	2.1
	Male	1,073	0.9	4.4	1,934	1.7
TOTAL		3,372	1.1	8.6	5,801	2.0

SOURCE: Vital Statistics of the United States

Figure 2. Diverticular Disease: Age-Adjusted Rates of Death in the United States, 1979–2004

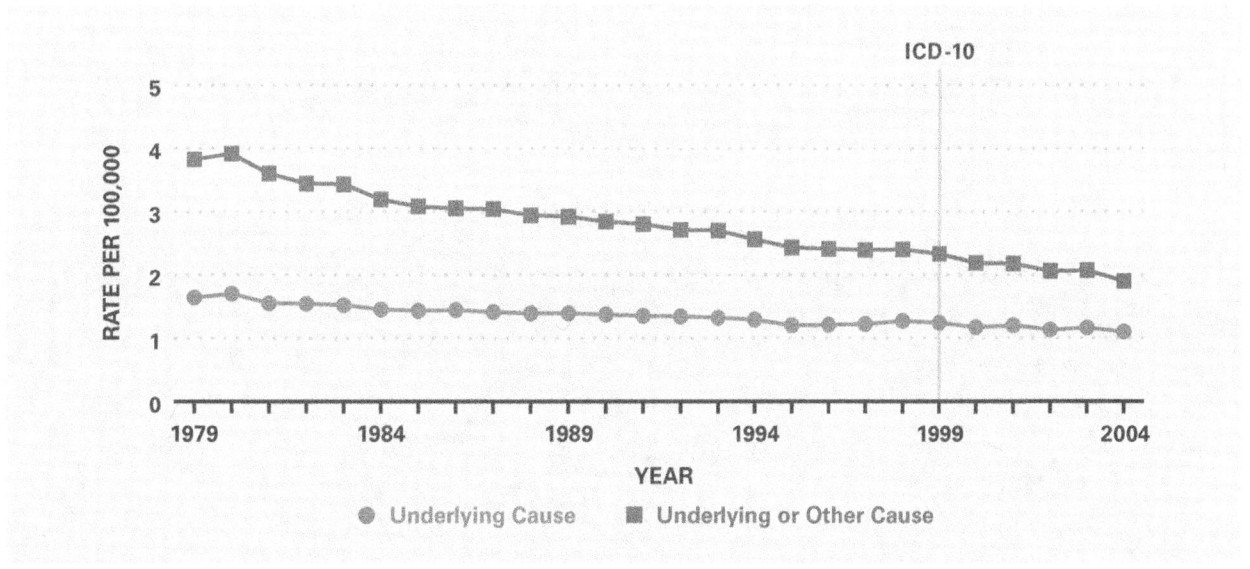

SOURCE: Vital Statistics of the United States

Table 3. Diverticular Disease: Costliest Prescriptions

DRUG	Prescription (#)	Prescription	Retail Cost	Cost
Ciprofloxacin	563,520	20.2%	$32,814,344	32.7%
Morphine	788,714	28.3	22,240,858	22.2
Levofloxacin	221,943	8.0	20,204,227	20.2
Metronidazole	745,223	26.7	11,416,565	11.4
Amoxicillin/Clavulanate	125,629	4.5	6,411,362	6.4
Hydrocodone/Acetaminophen	187,977	6.7	1,640,576	1.6
Oxycodone/Acetaminophen	47,534	1.7	1,190,000	1.2
Cephalexin	36,199	1.3	715,276	0.7
Ibuprofen/Hydrocodone	15,994	0.6	703,984	0.7
Moxifloxacin	5,577	0.2	611,465	0.6
Other	51,210	1.7	2,281,170	2.3
TOTAL	2,789,520	100.0%	$100,229,827	100.0%

SOURCE: Verispan

CHAPTER 21

Liver Disease

James E. Everhart, M.D., M.P.H.

There are many causes of liver disease, and the underlying cause is not always clear from administrative data sets. Thus, this report does not break out cause-specific liver disease other than viral hepatitis and hepatocellular carcinoma. Because ICD-10 does not separate acute from chronic liver disease, ICD-9 codes for acute and chronic liver disease were combined to achieve consistency for time trend data (Appendix 1).

In 2004, liver disease was the ninth leading diagnosis at ambulatory care visits, with 2.4 million visits (Table 1). If combined with the 3.5 million visits with a diagnosis of viral hepatitis, then liver disease would have been the third leading diagnosis, after GERD and chronic constipation. All-listed visit rates for liver disease were highest at age 45–64 years. Age-adjusted rates were higher for blacks than whites and slightly higher among females. When listed as a hospital discharge, liver disease was first-listed diagnosis on only 24.4 percent of records. In 2004, liver disease was the third leading diagnosis on hospital discharge records, after only GERD and diverticular disease. Combined with 475,000 viral hepatitis diagnoses, liver disease would have been the second leading diagnosis, with 1.2 million. Rates increased with age and were higher among blacks and males. The rates of age-adjusted ambulatory care visits increased steadily between 1992–1993 and 2003–2005 (Figure 1), in contrast to the 1970s and 1980s, when they were relatively constant.[1] Hospitalization rates were stable through the 1970s and fell throughout the 1980s, as was true for many other diseases.[2] Between 1999 and 2004, the rate of hospitalization with a diagnosis of liver disease increased by more than a third.

In 2004, there were 36,000 deaths with liver disease listed as underlying cause, which was half the number of deaths with liver disease listed as underlying or other cause (Table 2). Among all digestive diseases, liver disease was the second leading cause of death, after colorectal cancer. Death from liver disease was most common among persons aged 45–64 years, although the mortality rate from liver disease was highest at age 65 years and older. As a result of the large number of deaths occurring at an early age, the YPLL prior to age 75 years was higher than for any other digestive disease. Mortality rates were slightly higher among whites than blacks, and were nearly twice as high among males. Beginning in 1970, through 2004, mortality from liver disease declined slowly but steadily (Figure 2).[3] Between 1979 and 2004, liver disease mortality fell 30 percent. This rate of decline would have been halved had deaths from viral hepatitis been included.

According to the Verispan database of retail pharmacy prescriptions (Appendix 2), only three drugs (spironolactone, lactulose, and furosemide) were commonly prescribed for liver disease in 2004, for a total of 731,000 prescriptions at a cost of $16 million (Table 3). Spironolactone constituted 80 percent of both the number of prescriptions (583,000) and their cost ($12.8 million).

[1] Dufour MC. Chronic liver disease and cirrhosis. In: Everhart JE, editor. *Digestive diseases in the United States: epidemiology and impact*. US Department of Health and Human Services, Public Health Service, National Institutes of Health, National Institute of Diabetes and Digestive and Kidney Diseases. Washington, DC: US Government Printing Office, 1994; NIH Publication No. 94-1447 pp. 613–646.

[2] Ibid.

[3] Ibid.

Table 1. Liver Disease: Number and Age-Adjusted Rates of Ambulatory Care Visits and Hospital Discharges With First-Listed and All-Listed Diagnoses by Age, Race, and Sex in the United States, 2004

DEMOGRAPHIC CHARACTERISTICS		AMBULATORY CARE VISITS				HOSPITAL DISCHARGES			
		First-Listed Diagnosis		All-Listed Diagnoses		First-Listed Diagnosis		All-Listed Diagnoses	
		Number in Thousands	Rate per 100,000	Number in Thousands	Rate per 100,000	Number in Thousands	Rate per 100,000	Number in Thousands	Rate per 100,000
AGE (Years)	Under 15	—	—	—	—	2	2	9	14
	15–44	346	275	490	389	35	28	153	122
	45–64	665	941	1,374	1,944	102	144	365	517
	65+	358	986	503	1,385	47	129	233	640
RACE	White	1,122	446	1,903	749	149	59	596	236
	Black	198	654	289	912	21	63	96	292
SEX	Female	796	512	1,282	815	73	46	327	206
	Male	577	394	1,116	762	112	78	432	305
TOTAL		1,373	468	2,398	816	185	63	759	259

SOURCE: National Ambulatory Medical Care Survey (NAMCS) and National Hospital Ambulatory Medical Care Survey (NHAMCS) (3-year average, 2003–2005), and Healthcare Cost and Utilization Project Nationwide Inpatient Sample (HCUP NIS)

Figure 1. Liver Disease: Age-Adjusted Rates of Ambulatory Care Visits and Hospital Discharges With All-Listed Diagnoses in the United States, 1979–2004

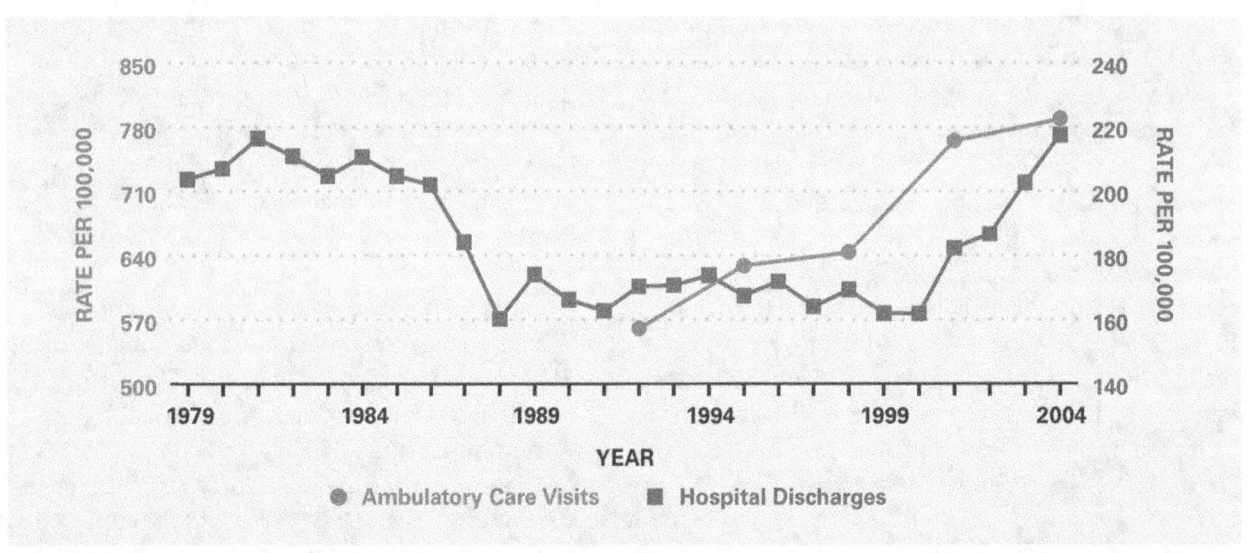

SOURCE: National Ambulatory Medical Care Survey (NAMCS) and National Hospital Ambulatory Medical Care Survey (NHAMCS) (averages 1992–1993, 1994–1996, 1997–1999, 2000–2002, 2003–2005), and National Hospital Discharge Survey (NHDS)

Table 2. Liver Disease: Number and Age-Adjusted Rates of Deaths and Years of Potential Life Lost (to Age 75) by Age, Race, and Sex in the United States, 2004

DEMOGRAPHIC CHARACTERISTICS		UNDERLYING CAUSE			UNDERLYING OR OTHER CAUSE	
		Number of Deaths	Rate per 100,000	Years of Potential Life Lost in Thousands	Number of Deaths	Rate per 100,000
AGE (Years)	Under 15	146	0.2	10.7	491	0.8
	15–44	4,169	3.3	146.4	7,851	6.2
	45–64	18,154	25.7	367.6	35,259	49.9
	65+	13,620	37.5	34.4	29,486	81.2
RACE	White	31,041	12.1	462.8	61,685	24.1
	Black	3,784	11.8	72.8	8,547	27.1
SEX	Female	13,385	8.2	178.9	27,503	16.8
	Male	22,705	16.2	380.2	45,588	32.8
TOTAL		36,090	12.3	559.1	73,091	24.9

SOURCE: Vital Statistics of the United States

Figure 2. Liver Disease: Age-Adjusted Rates of Death in the United States, 1979–2004

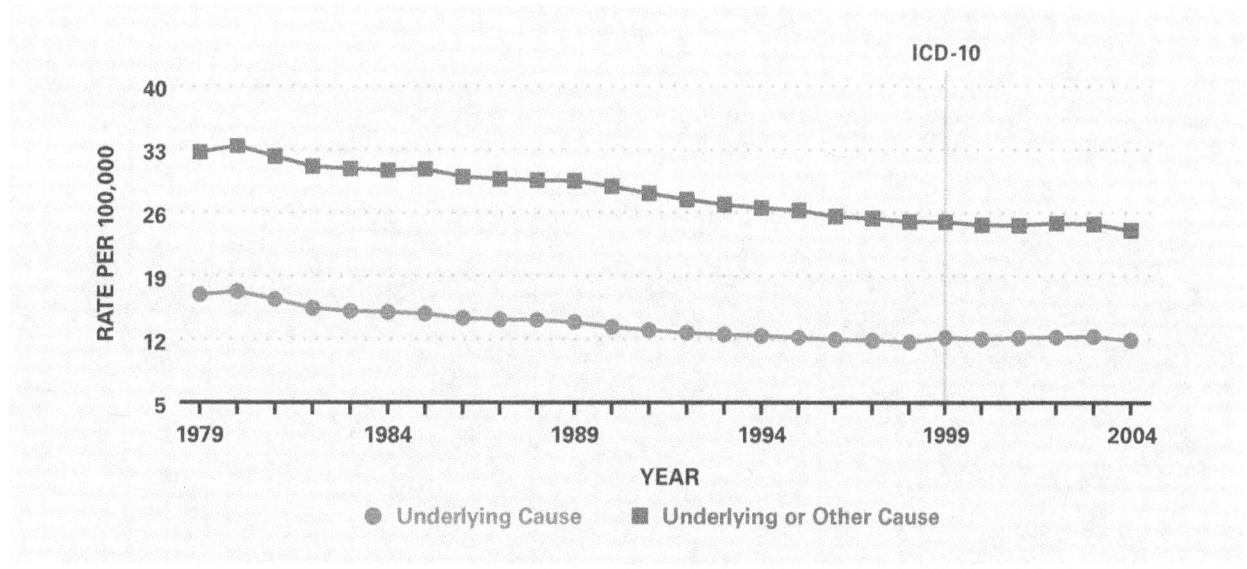

SOURCE: Vital Statistics of the United States

Table 3. Liver Disease: Costliest Prescriptions

DRUG	Prescription (#)	Prescription	Retail Cost	Cost
Spironolactone	583,486	79.8%	$12,838,400	80.0%
Lactulose	115,294	15.8	3,006,568	18.7
Furosemide	32,450	4.4	208,205	1.3
TOTAL	731,230	100.0%	$16,053,173	100.0%

SOURCE: Verispan

CHAPTER 22

Gallstones

James E. Everhart, M.D., M.P.H.

Gallstones (cholelithiasis) are coded with or without complications (choledocholithiasis, cholangitis, cholecystitis). Cholecystitis (inflammation of the gallbladder) without the presence of gallstones was not included (Appendix 1).

In 2004, there were an estimated 1.8 million ambulatory care visits with a diagnosis of gallstones, most of which were for gallstones as a first-listed diagnosis (Table 1). Visit rates increased with age, although only modestly after age 65 years. Age-adjusted rates for any visits were 18 percent higher among whites than blacks and 162 percent higher for females than males, which is in keeping with the known risks for gallstones. Gallstones ranked fifth among digestive diseases in all-listed discharge diagnoses in 2004. However, this was an underestimate of the actual hospital burden, because most hospitalizations with gallstones were for cholecystectomy, of which a high proportion were performed laparoscopically without overnight stay and, therefore, not included in hospitalization statistics.[1] Based on hospitalization rates prior to this shift in hospital care, gallstones would have ranked first among digestive diseases in first-listed diagnoses and second in all-listed (the first being GERD). Hospitalization rates with mention of gallstones increased with age, were similar for blacks and whites, and were 58 percent higher for women than men. Over time, rates of ambulatory care visits were relatively stable (Figure 1), but increased from the 1980s by at least 20 percent.[2] Hospitalization rates dropped by 40 percent in 2004 from their peak in 1991, because of the aforementioned change in hospital care.

Case-fatality rates for gallstones were low in 2004, but there were still more than 1,000 deaths with gallstones listed as underlying cause (Table 2), because the condition is so common and complications can be severe. The large majority of deaths occurred among persons age 65 years and older. Thus, there were only about 4 YPLL prior to age 75 years per death with gallstones as the underlying cause. Age-adjusted death rates differed little by race and by sex. Mortality rates fell between 1979 and 2004 by 56 percent for gallstones as underlying cause and by 71 percent as underlying or other cause (Figure 2). This was the greatest rate of decline for any common digestive disease, continuing a pattern from at least 1950, when more than 5,000 persons had gallstones listed as underlying cause of death.[3]

According to the Verispan database of retail pharmacy prescriptions (Appendix 2), in 2004, the total number of prescriptions for gallstones was 1.65 million at a retail cost of $18.6 million. Analgesics constituted more than 99 percent of these prescriptions.

[1] Everhart JE. Gallstones. In: Everhart JE, editor. *Digestive diseases in the United States: epidemiology and impact*. US Department of Health and Human Services, Public Health Service, National Institutes of Health, National Institute of Diabetes and Digestive and Kidney Diseases. Washington, DC: US Government Printing Office, 1994; NIH Publication No. 94-1447 pp. 647–690.

[2] Ibid.

[3] Ibid.

Table 1. Gallstones: Number and Age-Adjusted Rates of Ambulatory Care Visits and Hospital Discharges With First-Listed and All-Listed Diagnoses by Age, Race, and Sex in the United States, 2004

		AMBULATORY CARE VISITS				HOSPITAL DISCHARGES			
		First-Listed Diagnosis		All-Listed Diagnoses		First-Listed Diagnosis		All-Listed Diagnoses	
DEMOGRAPHIC CHARACTERISTICS		Number in Thousands	Rate per 100,000	Number in Thousands	Rate per 100,000	Number in Thousands	Rate per 100,000	Number in Thousands	Rate per 100,000
AGE (Years)	Under 15	—	—	—	—	2	4	4	6
	15–44	443	352	651	518	119	95	179	142
	45–64	522	739	734	1,039	106	150	180	255
	65+	321	883	411	1,132	124	341	259	713
RACE	White	1,041	421	1,516	615	278	112	490	195
	Black	127	369	179	521	34	102	63	198
SEX	Female	932	604	1,358	882	235	151	406	256
	Male	367	260	478	336	114	85	214	162
TOTAL		1,299	442	1,836	625	352	120	622	212

SOURCE: National Ambulatory Medical Care Survey (NAMCS) and National Hospital Ambulatory Medical Care Survey (NHAMCS) (3-year average, 2003–2005), and Healthcare Cost and Utilization Project Nationwide Inpatient Sample (HCUP NIS)

Figure 1. Gallstones: Age-Adjusted Rates of Ambulatory Care Visits and Hospital Discharges With All-Listed Diagnoses in the United States, 1979–2004

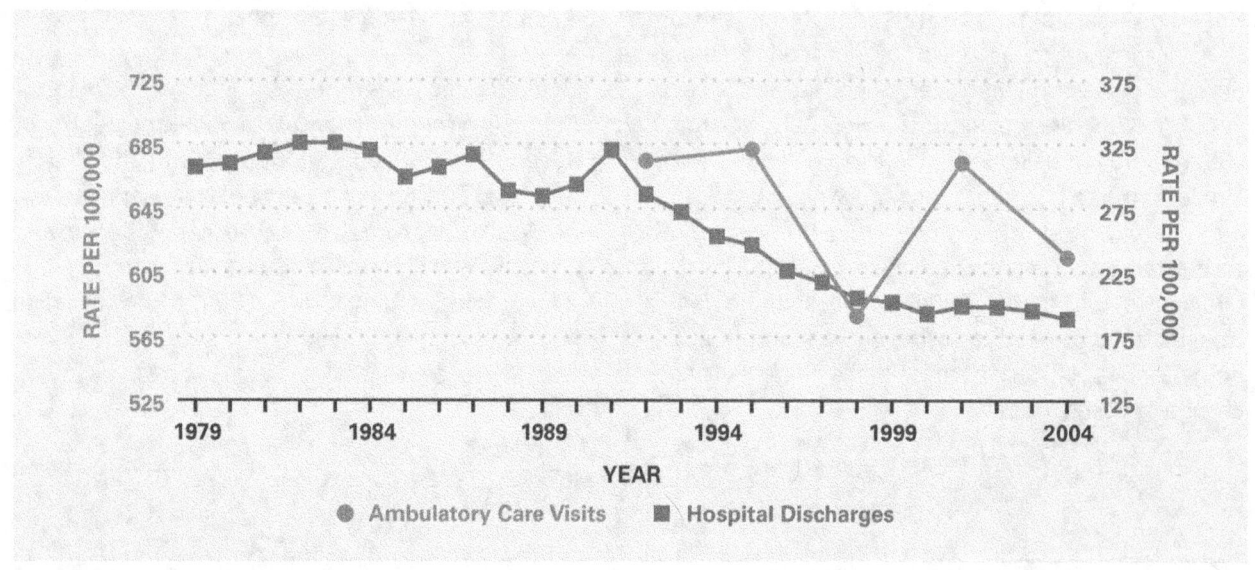

SOURCE: National Ambulatory Medical Care Survey (NAMCS) and National Hospital Ambulatory Medical Care Survey (NHAMCS) (averages 1992–1993, 1994–1996, 1997–1999, 2000–2002, 2003–2005), and National Hospital Discharge Survey (NHDS)

Table 2. Gallstones: Number and Age-Adjusted Rates of Deaths and Years of Potential Life Lost (to Age 75) by Age, Race, and Sex in the United States, 2004

DEMOGRAPHIC CHARACTERISTICS		UNDERLYING CAUSE			UNDERLYING OR OTHER CAUSE	
		Number of Deaths	Rate per 100,000	Years of Potential Life Lost in Thousands	Number of Deaths	Rate per 100,000
AGE (Years)	Under 15	—	—	—	1	0.0
	15–44	31	0.0	1.1	75	0.1
	45–64	137	0.2	2.6	276	0.4
	65+	924	2.5	0.6	1,803	5.0
RACE	White	960	0.4	3.3	1,883	0.7
	Black	90	0.3	0.7	199	0.8
SEX	Female	648	0.3	2.0	1,256	0.7
	Male	444	0.4	2.4	899	0.8
TOTAL		1,092	0.4	4.4	2,155	0.7

SOURCE: Vital Statistics of the United States

Figure 2. Gallstones: Age-Adjusted Rates of Death in the United States, 1979–2004

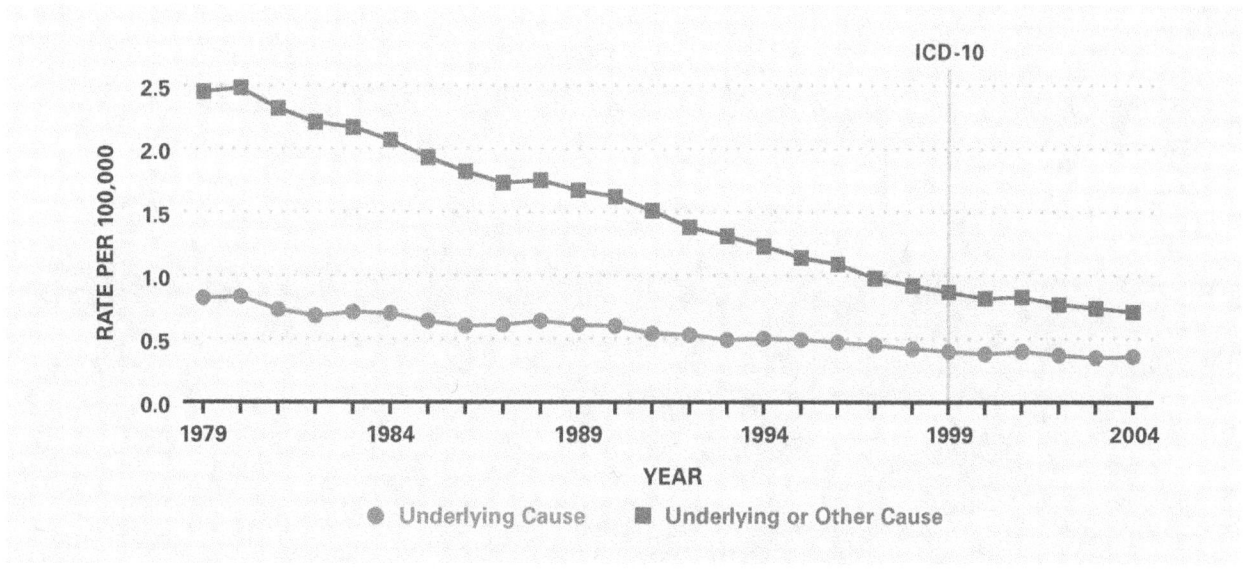

SOURCE: Vital Statistics of the United States

CHAPTER 23

Pancreatitis

James E. Everhart, M.D., M.P.H.

Pancreatitis is coded as acute or chronic, and the two are grouped together in this chapter, although acute pancreatitis has the greater burden of medical care and mortality.[1] In 2004, there were 475,000 ambulatory care visits as first-listed diagnosis and 881,000 visits as all-listed diagnoses (Table 1). Rates of visits with pancreatitis as all-listed diagnoses increased moderately with age. Age-adjusted rates were 25 percent higher among blacks than whites and 52 percent higher among females than males. Pancreatitis was the seventh most commonly noted digestive disease diagnosis on hospitalization, just after peptic ulcer disease. Hospitalization rates increased with age and were 88 percent higher among blacks and 11 percent higher among males. Rates of both ambulatory care visits and hospitalizations with pancreatitis increased from the 1980s to 2004 (Figure 1). In particular, the rate of hospital discharges with a pancreatitis diagnosis increased 62 percent between 1988 and 2004.

In 2004, pancreatitis was the eleventh most common underlying cause of death from digestive diseases and the fifth most common nonmalignant cause, just after peptic ulcer disease. More than half of deaths occurred among persons age 65 years and older (Table 2).

Pancreatitis ranked eighth among all digestive diseases in YPLL prior to age 75, with about 43,000 years or 12.3 years per death. Death rates increased with age and were higher among blacks than whites and men than women. Mortality rates fell slightly from 1979 to 2004 (Figure 2), with the rate for underlying cause having fallen 15 percent over this 25-year period.

According to the Verispan database of retail pharmacy prescriptions (Appendix 2), in 2004, the total number of prescriptions for pancreatitis was approximately 766,000 at a retail cost of roughly $88.6 million (Table 3). Pancreatic enzyme replacements constituted 60.3 percent of the prescriptions and 84.8 percent of the cost. All the other prescriptions were analgesics or antiemetic agents.

[1] Go VLW, Everhart JE. Pancreatitis. In: Everhart JE, editor. *Digestive diseases in the United States: epidemiology and impact*. US Department of Health and Human Services, Public Health Service, National Institutes of Health, National Institute of Diabetes and Digestive and Kidney Diseases. Washington, DC: US Government Printing Office, 1994; NIH Publication No. 94-1447 pp. 691–712.

Table 1. Pancreatitis: Number and Age-Adjusted Rates of Ambulatory Care Visits and Hospital Discharges With First-Listed and All-Listed Diagnoses by Age, Race, and Sex in the United States, 2004

DEMOGRAPHIC CHARACTERISTICS		AMBULATORY CARE VISITS				HOSPITAL DISCHARGES			
		First-Listed Diagnosis		All-Listed Diagnoses		First-Listed Diagnosis		All-Listed Diagnoses	
		Number in Thousands	Rate per 100,000	Number in Thousands	Rate per 100,000	Number in Thousands	Rate per 100,000	Number in Thousands	Rate per 100,000
AGE (Years)	Under 15	—	—	—	—	3	5	5	8
	15–44	153	121	304	241	99	78	152	120
	45–64	219	310	354	500	104	147	171	242
	65+	101	279	222	611	72	197	127	349
RACE	White	396	160	721	294	194	78	318	128
	Black	77	213	129	368	46	136	81	241
SEX	Female	306	199	545	355	136	87	228	145
	Male	169	116	336	234	140	100	226	161
TOTAL		475	162	881	300	277	94	454	155

SOURCE: National Ambulatory Medical Care Survey (NAMCS) and National Hospital Ambulatory Medical Care Survey (NHAMCS) (3-year average, 2003–2005), and Healthcare Cost and Utilization Project Nationwide Inpatient Sample (HCUP NIS)

Figure 1. Pancreatitis: Age-Adjusted Rates of Ambulatory Care Visits and Hospital Discharges With All-Listed Diagnoses in the United States, 1979–2004

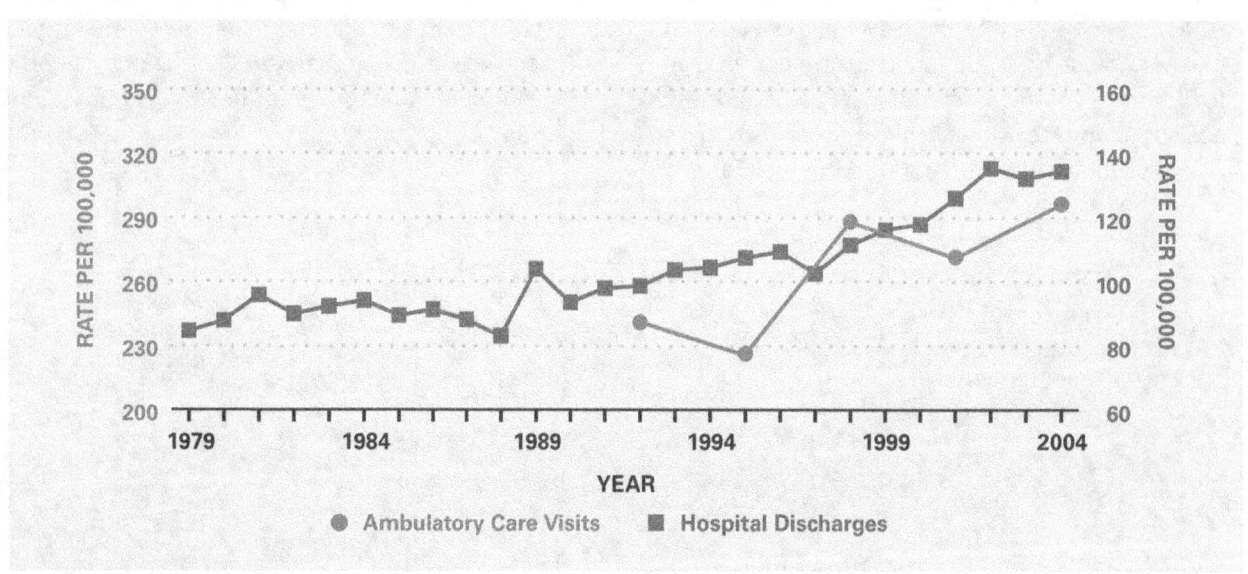

SOURCE: National Ambulatory Medical Care Survey (NAMCS) and National Hospital Ambulatory Medical Care Survey (NHAMCS) (averages 1992–1993, 1994–1996, 1997–1999, 2000–2002, 2003–2005), and National Hospital Discharge Survey (NHDS)

Table 2. Pancreatitis: Number and Age-Adjusted Rates of Deaths and Years of Potential Life Lost (to Age 75) by Age, Race, and Sex in the United States, 2004

DEMOGRAPHIC CHARACTERISTICS		UNDERLYING CAUSE			UNDERLYING OR OTHER CAUSE	
		Number of Deaths	Rate per 100,000	Years of Potential Life Lost in Thousands	Number of Deaths	Rate per 100,000
AGE (Years)	Under 15	15	0.0	1.0	26	0.0
	15–44	467	0.4	17.8	888	0.7
	45–64	1,044	1.5	21.0	2,222	3.1
	65+	1,953	5.4	3.0	4,005	11.0
RACE	White	2,838	1.1	31.7	5,739	2.2
	Black	557	1.8	9.7	1,210	4.0
SEX	Female	1,549	0.9	13.0	3,239	1.9
	Male	1,931	1.5	29.8	3,903	3.0
TOTAL		3,480	1.2	42.8	7,142	2.4

SOURCE: Vital Statistics of the United States

Figure 2. Pancreatitis: Age-Adjusted Rates of Death in the United States, 1979–2004

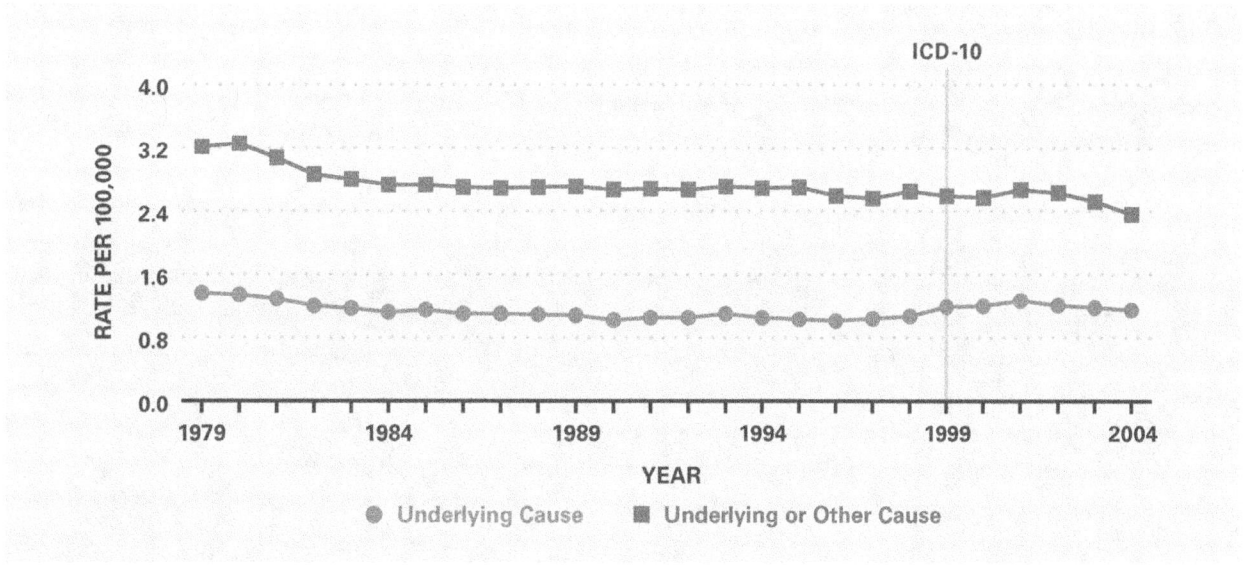

SOURCE: Vital Statistics of the United States

Table 3. Pancreatitis: Costliest Prescriptions

DRUG	Prescription (#)	Prescription	Retail Cost	Cost
Amylase/Lipase/Protease	343,519	44.8%	$54,085,858	61.1%
Pancrelipase	118,277	15.4	21,041,841	23.8
Hydrocodone/Acetaminophen	171,121	22.3	6,524,330	7.4
Oxycodone/Acetaminophen	76,199	9.9	3,970,182	4.5
Oxycodone	25,097	3.3	2,629,763	3.0
Promethazine	20,846	2.7	184,599	0.2
Codeine/Acetaminophen	8,808	1.1	89,625	0.1
Acetyl Salicylic Acid/Oxycodone	964	0.1	30,971	0.0
Meperidine	1,139	0.1	21,709	0.0
Prochlorperazine	394	0.0	3,834	0.0
TOTAL	766,364	100.0%	$88,582,712	100.0%

SOURCE: Verispan

CHAPTER 24

Indications and Outcomes of Gastrointestinal Endoscopy

Constance E. Ruhl, M.D., Ph.D.; and James E. Everhart, M.D., M.P.H.

Through diagnosis and management, endoscopy plays a role in nearly all GI diseases as well as a crucial role in clinical research. It is estimated that more than 20 million GI endoscopies are performed yearly in the United States.[1] There is no single national endoscopic database that can provide accurate population-based information on the absolute number of GI endoscopies and their indications and diagnostic outcomes. To remedy this important gap in knowledge on the burden of GI disease, data were obtained from the Clinical Outcomes Research Initiative's (CORI) National Endoscopic Database (NED). For more than 10 years, this project has collected and analyzed computerized endoscopic records gathered from diverse endoscopic practices throughout the United States. Pediatric procedures are not represented, and the participating sites are overrepresented by veteran and military facilities. Nevertheless, the patterns of endoscopy in NED have been shown to be quite similar to that of a national sample of the Medicare population and may well be applicable to the United States as a whole.[2] There is no independent confirmation of the indications and diagnoses reported by the endoscopist on the endoscopy record, although the report is frequently included in the medical record and used for billing.

For this report, endoscopic data were obtained for the period 2001–2005. The number of patients receiving the various endoscopic procedures, along with the practices and practice sites where the procedures were conducted, is shown in Table 1. Of the 885,593 procedures performed during this period, 61.2 percent were colonoscopies, 30.6 percent were esophagogastroduodenoscopies (EGD), 6.3 percent were flexible sigmoidoscopies, 1.0 percent were endoscopic retrograde cholangiopancreatography (ERCP), and 0.8 percent were endoscopic ultrasonographies (EUS). Colonoscopy, flexible sigmoidoscopy, and EGD were primarily performed within community or health maintenance organization (HMO) practices in hospital or ambulatory surgery centers. The more specialized procedures of ERCP and EUS were more likely to have been performed in academic centers and almost exclusively in the hospital. Age 50–59 years was the peak age group for all the procedures. There was some ethnic variation in likelihood of receiving a particular procedure, relative to all procedures. Non-Hispanic whites were more likely to have undergone colonoscopy (85.9 percent) and EUS (86.9 percent), non-Hispanic blacks (13.3 percent) and Asian-Pacific Islanders (2.2 percent) flexible sigmoidoscopy, and Native Americans (6.0 percent) and Hispanics (12.4 percent) ERCP. Excluding Veterans Affairs (VA) facilities, the majority of procedures were performed on women.

Of the 101 sites providing data to NED during 2001–2005, 36 did so throughout the 5-year period. At these "stable" sites, the total number of procedures increased by 34.1 percent from 2001 to 2005, but trends differed by procedure (Figure 1). Colonoscopy increased 63.4 percent, partly at the expense of flexible sigmoidoscopy, which decreased by 60.0 percent. EGD increased by 20.3 percent. The frequency of each of these procedures peaked at age 50–59 years, but more so for colonoscopy (Figure 2). At the stable sites, the growth in colonoscopy from 2001 to 2005 was concentrated among this age group and to a lesser extent among persons ages 60–69 years (Figure 3). The number of colonoscopies among other age groups changed little. In contrast, the number of sigmoidoscopies at stable sites declined appreciably among persons ages 40–79 years, but most among those ages 50–79 (Figure 4).

The distribution of indications for all colonoscopies and sigmoidoscopies is shown in Table 2. Because there could be more than one indication for a procedure, the totals of the percentages exceeded 100 percent. Broadly speaking, surveillance and symptoms were more often listed as indications for colonoscopy than for sigmoidoscopy, while screening was a more frequent indication for sigmoidoscopy than for colonoscopy. Suspected bleeding was the most common indication for colonoscopy (29.7 percent), followed by screening of persons at routine risk of colorectal cancer (21.6 percent), surveillance of adenomatous polyps (13.5 percent), and screening for persons with a family history of colorectal cancer (12.1 percent). These most common indications for colonoscopy indicate that concern over possible colorectal cancer was the predominant reason for colonoscopy. The same statement can be made for sigmoidoscopy, except that a high percentage (47.4 percent) were performed for persons at routine risk of colorectal cancer.

The findings among persons who had colonoscopies or sigmoidoscopies are shown in Table 3. The most interesting group is the column of colonoscopic findings among persons at routine risk only, among whom findings should not have been influenced by symptoms or other indications for the procedure. As long as all abnormalities were recorded, these may be considered the prevalence of such findings in the general population. Common but benign conditions such as diverticulosis and hemorrhoids may not have been recorded if a more serious problem was diagnosed. Notably, 21.0 percent of examinations were normal and 6.4 percent found a polyp of at least 1 centimeter or a suspected malignancy. Figure 5 demonstrates colonoscopic findings among persons at routine risk according to age group. Diverticulosis, the most common finding, steadily increased in prevalence from age 50–59 years to age 80 years and older, at which point it was found on 71.4 percent of examinations. Increasing in prevalence with age, but not as quickly as diverticulosis, were polyps of all sizes and number, and hemorrhoids. The prevalence of normal examinations fell from 36.2 percent at age 20–39 years to 10.2 percent at 80 years and above. There was a higher prevalence of polyps among men than women at routine risk (Figure 6), but no other particular differences by sex. Hemorrhoids were more common among Hispanics, but no other racial or ethnic differences were evident (Figure 7).

In contrast to the uneven increase in utilization of colonoscopy across age groups, EGD use increased modestly across all age groups at stable sites (Figure 8). The indications for EGD at all NED sites are shown in Table 4. These indications were not mutually exclusive and included groupings of symptoms, notably alarm symptoms (weight loss, vomiting, or bleeding) and bleeding (anemia, iron deficiency, melena, hematemesis, hematochezia, positive fecal occult blood test, or suspected upper GI bleed). The most common indications for EGD were reflux symptoms (28.3 percent), alarm symptoms (27.7 percent), dysphagia (20.5 percent), signs of bleeding (20.4 percent), and abdominal pain or bloating (20.1 percent). More than 40 percent of examinations had normal findings (Table 5). The most common diagnostic abnormalities were mucosal abnormality, hiatal hernia, and esophageal inflammation, each of which is characteristic of GERD. The next three most common diagnoses, stricture/stenosis, Barrett's esophagus, and ulcer, can be consequences of GERD. Combining these diagnoses, it can be inferred that the large majority of abnormal findings on EGD are associated with GERD.

ERCP findings from 2001–2005 are shown in Table 6. Because there were fewer than 10,000 ERCP reports from relatively few centers, the generalizability of the results is questionable. Also, some important information appeared in free text fields in the report, making interpretation more difficult. Nevertheless, it appeared that ductal abnormalities and obstruction to flow were the most common findings on ERCP, and that one-third of examinations were normal. EUS was performed too infrequently and at too few sites to present information on either indication or results.

[1] Seeff LC, Richards TB, Shapiro JA, Nadel MR, Manninen DL, Given LS, Dong FB, Winges LD, McKenna MT. How many endoscopies are performed for colorectal cancer screening? Results from CDC's survey of endoscopic capacity. *Gastroenterology.* 2004;127:1670–1677.

[2] Sonnenberg A, Amorosi SL, Lacey MJ, Lieberman DA. Patterns of endoscopy in the United States: analysis of data from the Centers for Medicare and Medicaid Services and the National Endoscopic Database. *Gastrointestinal endoscopy.* 2008;67:489–496.

Table 1. Characteristics of Endoscopy Sites and Persons Undergoing Endoscopic Procedures, 2001–2005

		COLONOSCOPY	EGD	FLEXIBLE SIGMOIDOSCOPY	ERCP	EUS
Number of Patients		542,650	270,957	55,708	9,333	6,945
Number of Practices		76	77	72	40	23
Number of Sites		101	101	96	44	25
SITE CHARACTERISTICS (Percentage)						
TYPE OF ENDOSCOPY SITE	Community/HMO	78.1	72.8	58.5	40.1	2.9
	Academic	11.3	14.6	16.6	41.1	66.5
	VA/Military	10.6	12.6	24.9	18.8	30.6
TYPE OF FACILITY	Office	1.7	2.7	1.1	<0.1	0
	Hospital	40.9	49.7	51.3	96.7	100
	Ambulatory Surgery Center	57.4	47.6	47.7	3.3	<0.1
PATIENT CHARACTERISTICS (Percentage)						
AGE (Years)	20–29	1.7	4.6	5.6	9.2	2.3
	30–39	4.0	9.4	8.6	10.3	5.3
	40–49	11.7	17.4	12.2	14.1	13.1
	50–59	32.9	23.1	34.6	19.3	24.3
	60–69	25.6	19.5	19.8	16.5	24.1
	70–79	18.4	17.5	13.6	18.3	22.8
	80+	5.9	8.6	5.6	12.4	8.1
RACE/ETHNICITY	Non-Hispanic White	85.9	81.3	78.2	72.0	86.9
	Non-Hispanic Black	6.4	7.3	13.3	7.5	5.0
	Asian/Pacific Islander	1.5	2.0	2.2	1.8	1.8
	American Indian/Alaska Native	0.8	1.2	0.9	6.0	0.4
	Multiracial Non-Hispanic	0.2	0.2	0.6	0.3	0.3
	Hispanic	5.3	8.0	4.8	12.4	5.6
SEX	Female	49.6	51.4	41.0	52.0	40.7
	Male	50.4	48.6	59.0	48.0	59.3
SEX (Excluding VA/Military)	Number of Patients	485,085	236,848	41,839	7,577	4,819
	Female	54.3	57.2	52.7	61.1	51.6
	Male	45.8	42.8	47.3	38.9	48.4

EGD = Esophagogastroduodenoscopy; ERCP = Endoscopic retrograde cholangiopancreatography; EUS = Endoscopic ultrasonography; VA = Department of Veterans Affairs
SOURCE: National Endoscopy Database/Clinical Outcomes Research Initiative

Figure 1. Number of Endoscopic Procedures at Stable Sites (N=36) by Year, 2001–2005

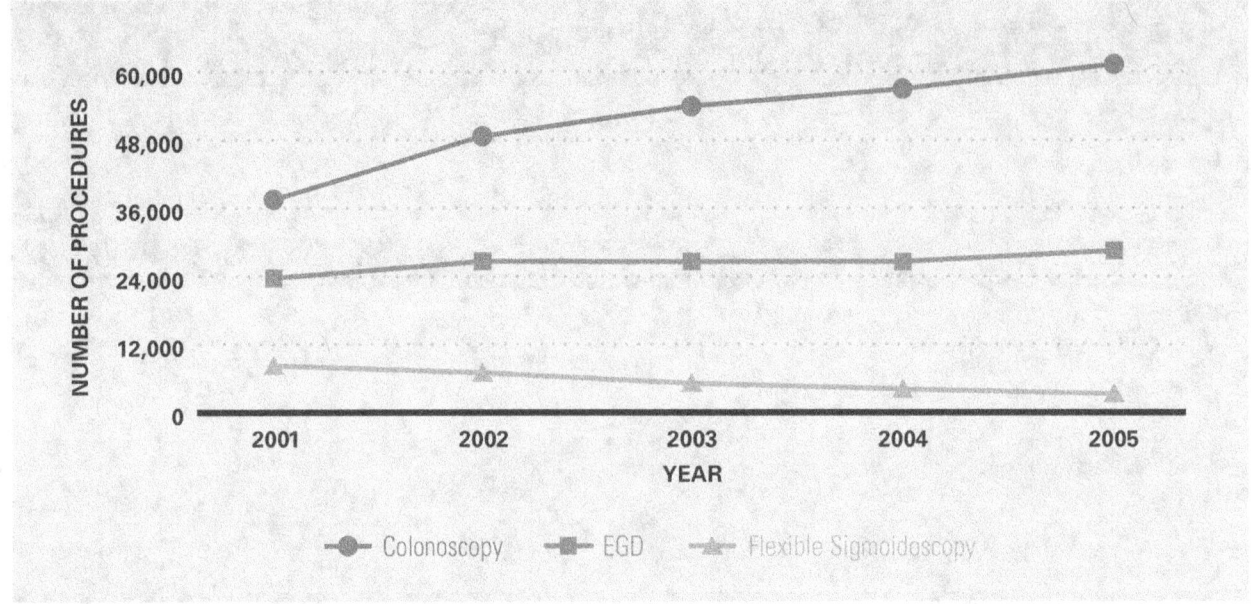

EGD = Esophagogastroduodenoscopy
SOURCE: National Endoscopy Database/Clinical Outcomes Research Initiative

Figure 2. Number of Endoscopic Procedures by Age, 2001–2005

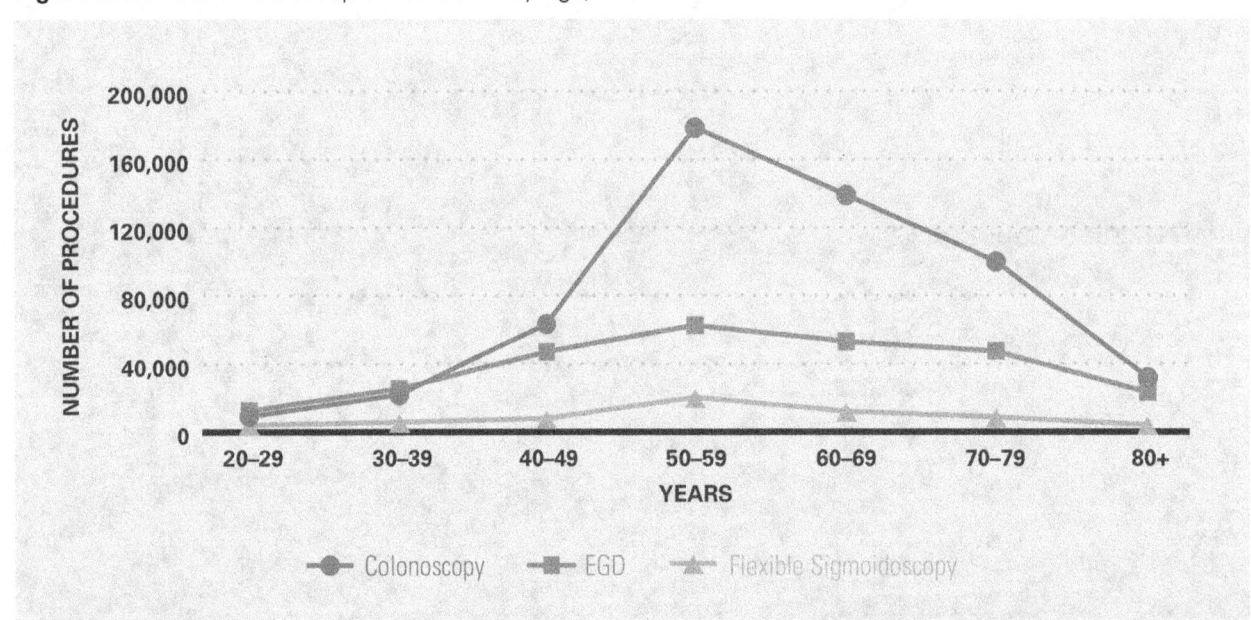

EGD = Esophagogastroduodenoscopy
SOURCE: National Endoscopy Database/Clinical Outcomes Research Initiative

Figure 3. Number of Colonoscopies at Stable Sites (N=36) by Age and Year, 2001–2005

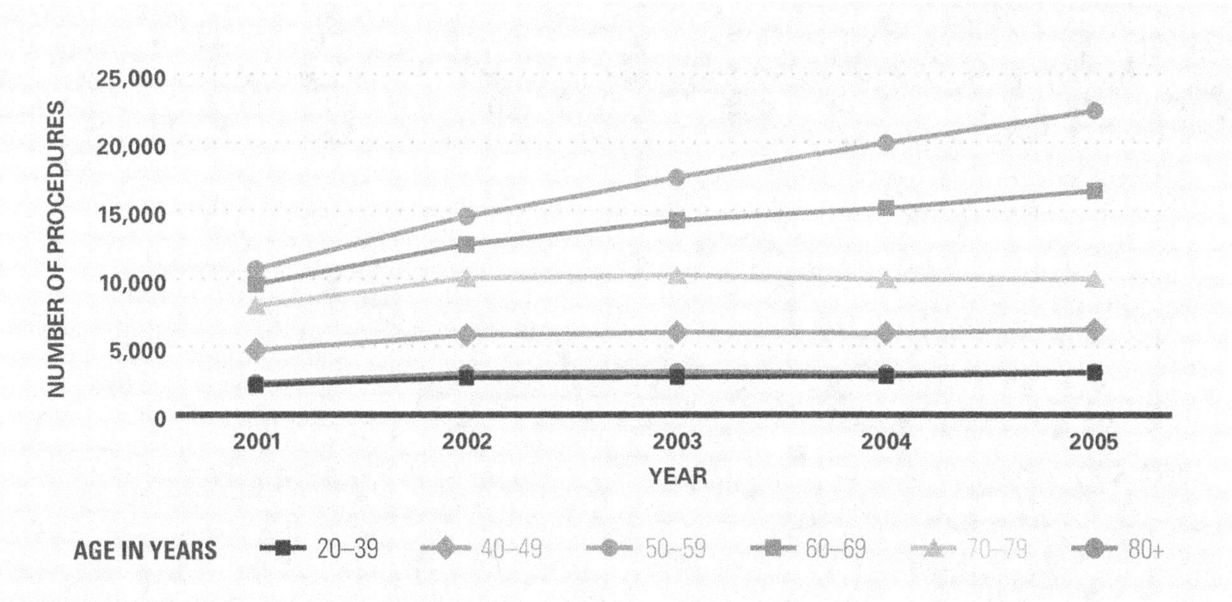

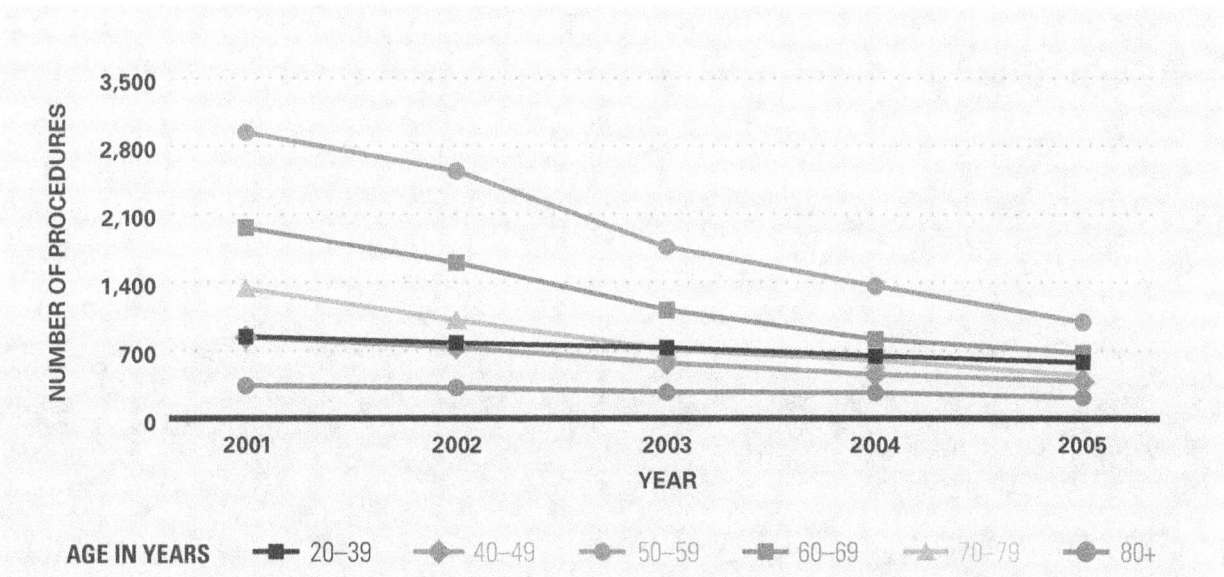

SOURCE: National Endoscopy Database/Clinical Outcomes Research Initiative

Figure 4. Number of Flexible Sigmoidoscopies at Stable Sites (N=36) by Age and Year, 2001–2005

SOURCE: National Endoscopy Database/Clinical Outcomes Research Initiative

Table 2. Indications for Colonoscopy and Flexible Sigmoidoscopy, 2001–2005

		PERCENTAGE[1]	
INDICATION		COLONOSCOPY (N=542,650)	FLEXIBLE SIGMOIDOSCOPY (N=55,708)
SURVEILLANCE	Surveillance of Adenomatous Polyps	13.5	2.4
	Surveillance of Colorectal Cancer	2.0	1.0
	Surveillance of Ulcerative Colitis	0.9	1.0
	Surveillance of Crohn's Disease	0.6	0.4
	Established Crohn's Disease	0.2	0.2
	Established Ulcerative Colitis	0.2	0.6
SCREENING	Routine Risk Only	21.6	47.4
	Family History of Colorectal Cancer	12.1	1.0
	Family History of Polyps	2.8	0.3
SYMPTOMS	Bleeding Group[2]	29.7	21.7
	Irritable Bowel Syndrome Cluster[3]	18.2	15.0
	Hematochezia	17.9	20.4
	Abdominal Pain/Bloating	9.1	5.4
	Diarrhea	7.6	9.9
	Positive Fecal Occult Blood Test	7.2	0.7
	Change in Bowel Habits	7.1	1.6
	Anemia	5.7	0.9
	Constipation	5.4	4.5
	Weight Loss	1.6	0.5
	Melena	0.7	0.2
	Iron Deficiency Without Anemia	0.3	< 0.1
FOLLOWUP OF DIAGNOSIS	Polyp Found on Flexible Sigmoidoscopy	1.5	0.2
	Abnormal Study	1.0	1.2
	History of Non-Gastrointestinal Cancer	0.8	0.3
	Suspected Inflammatory Bowel Disease	0.5	0.6
	Polyp Found on Barium Enema	0.2	0.1
	Polyp Found on Previous Colonoscopy	0.2	0.4
OTHER		6.5	11.5

[1] Indication categories are not mutually exclusive.

[2] Bleeding group = one or more of the following symptoms: anemia or iron deficiency, positive fecal occult blood test, hematochezia, melena.

[3] Irritable bowel syndrome cluster = one or more of the following symptoms: diarrhea; constipation; abdominal pain/bloating; change in bowel habits, excluding surveillance of, or established Crohn's disease or ulcerative colitis; weight loss; and bleeding (anemia or iron deficiency, positive fecal occult blood test, hematochezia, melena).

SOURCE: National Endoscopy Database/Clinical Outcomes Research Initiative

Table 3. Colonoscopy Findings in the Total Population and Persons at Routine Risk Only, and Flexible Sigmoidoscopy Findings, 2001–2005

| | PERCENTAGE[1] | | |
| | COLONOSCOPY | | FLEXIBLE SIGMOIDOSCOPY (N=55,708) |
FINDING	Total Population (N=542,650)	Routine Risk Only (N=117,422)	
Diverticulosis	42.8	45.0	22.3
Hemorrhoids	39.6	34.2	31.7
Polyp	35.9	37.4	16.2
Normal Exam/No Findings	17.6	21.0	30.5
Polyp > 9mm/Suspected Malignant Tumor	7.6	6.4	3.4
Multiple Polyps	7.2	7.2	2.8
Mucosal Abnormality-Colitis	5.2	1.4	7.8
Tumor	1.2	0.4	0.9
Angiodysplasia (AVM)	1.1	0.7	0.3
Other Finding	9.8	6.6	12.1

AVM = arteriovenous malformation

[1] Finding categories are not mutually exclusive.

SOURCE: National Endoscopy Database/Clinical Outcomes Research Initiative

Figure 5. Colonoscopy Findings in Persons at Routine Risk by Age, 2001–2005

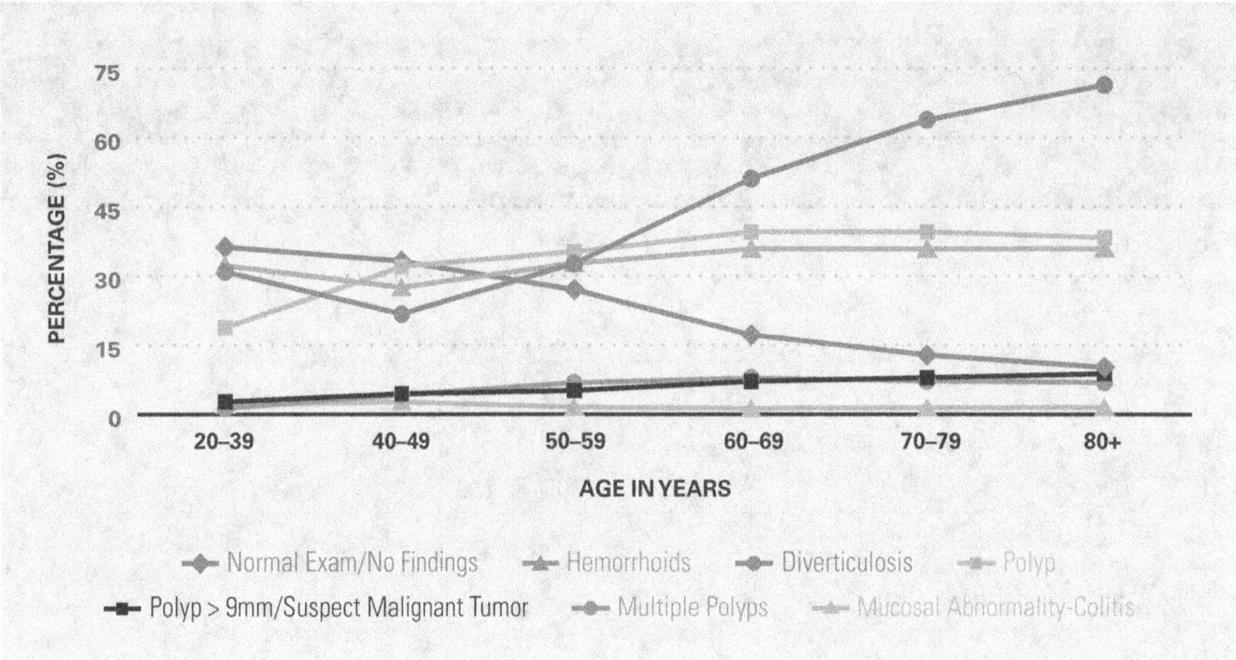

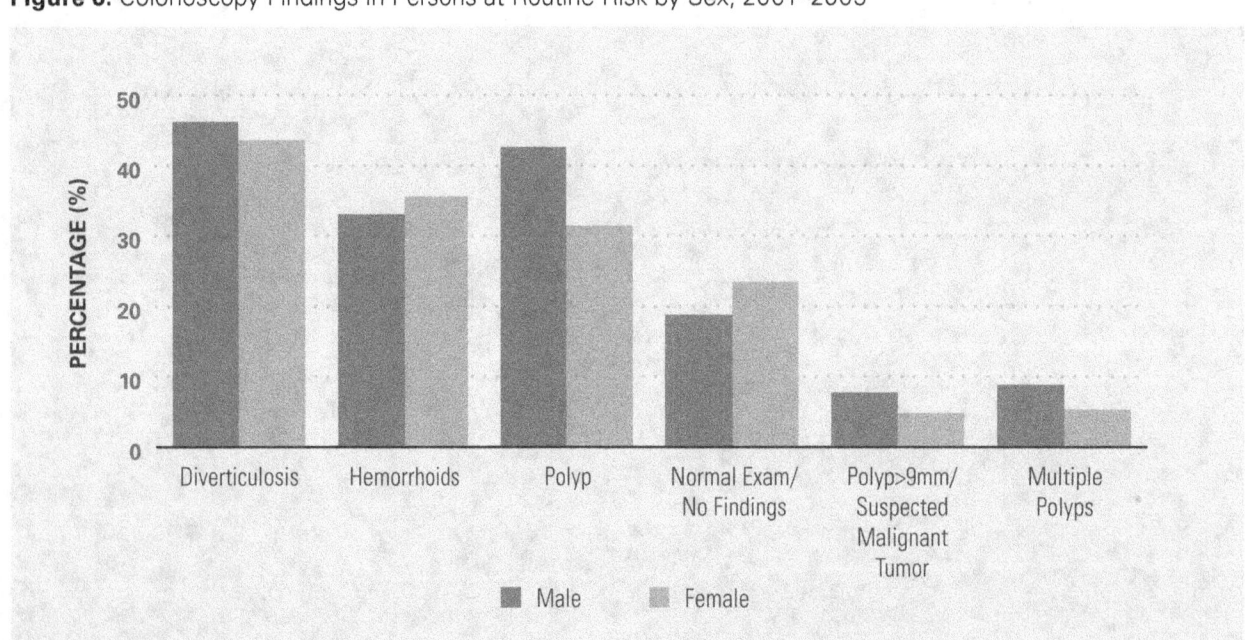

SOURCE: National Endoscopy Database/Clinical Outcomes Research Initiative

Figure 6. Colonoscopy Findings in Persons at Routine Risk by Sex, 2001–2005

SOURCE: National Endoscopy Database/Clinical Outcomes Research Initiative

Figure 7. Colonoscopy Findings in Persons at Routine Risk by Race/Ethnicity, 2001–2005

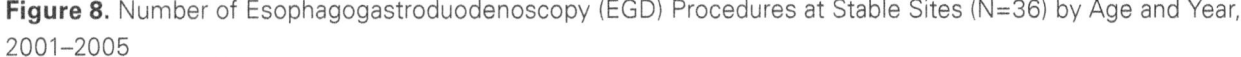

SOURCE: National Endoscopy Database/Clinical Outcomes Research Initiative

Figure 8. Number of Esophagogastroduodenoscopy (EGD) Procedures at Stable Sites (N=36) by Age and Year, 2001–2005

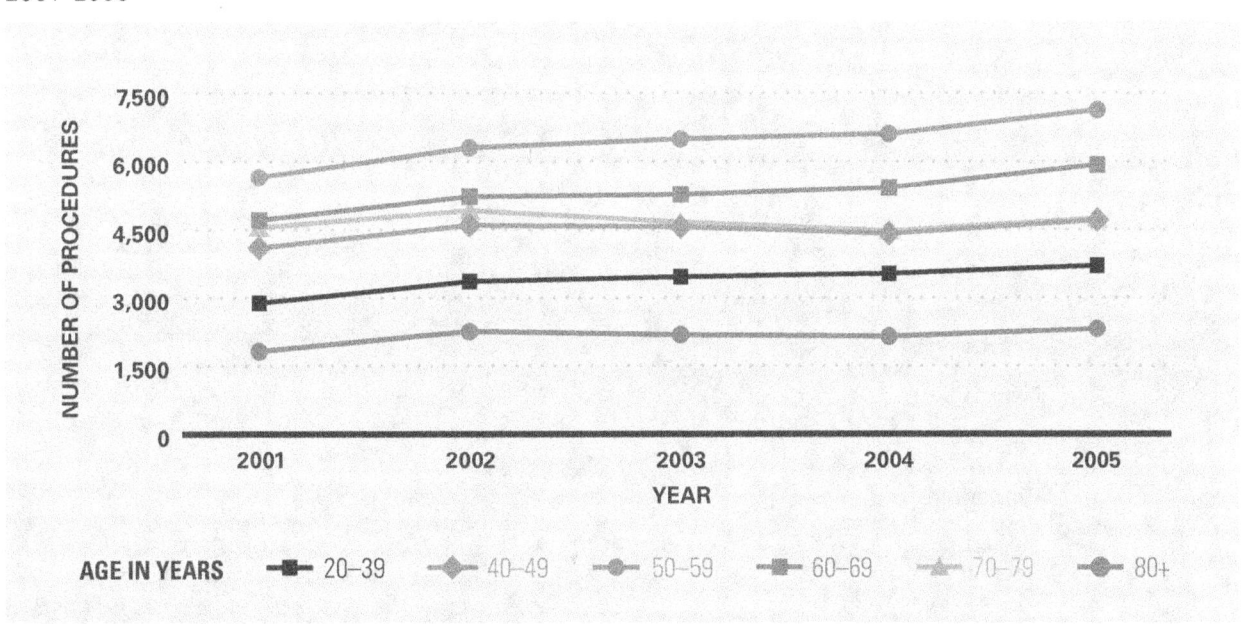

EGD = Esophagogastroduodenoscopy
SOURCE: National Endoscopy Database/Clinical Outcomes Research Initiative

Table 4. Indications for Esophagogastroduodenoscopy (EGD) (N=270,957), 2001–2005

INDICATION		PERCENTAGE[1]
SURVEILLANCE	Surveillance of Barrett's Esophagus	3.1
	Surveillance of Gastric Ulcer	1.0
	Surveillance of Varices	0.9
	Surveillance of *Helicobacter Pylori*	0.3
	Surveillance of Duodenal Ulcer	0.2
	Surveillance of Gastric Polyps	0.2
SCREENING	Screening for Barrett's Esophagus	1.5
	Screening for Varices	0.9
SYMPTOMS	Reflux Symptoms/Heartburn	28.3
	Alarm Symptoms[2]	27.7
	GERD[3]	22.3
	Dyspepsia/Abdominal Pain[4]	21.6
	Dysphagia	20.5
	Bleeding Cluster[5]	20.4
	Abdominal Pain/Bloating	20.1
	Anemia	10.5
	Dyspepsia	9.7
	Nausea	6.7
	Vomiting	4.9
	Melena	4.6
	Weight Loss	4.0
	Chest Pain	3.9
	Hematemesis	2.8
	Diarrhea	2.4
	Early Satiety	1.3
	Hematochezia	0.9
	Anorexia	0.8
	Odynophagia	0.7
	Pulmonary Symptoms	0.7
	Iron Deficiency Without Anemia	0.5
	Malabsorption	0.2
	Feeding Refusal	0.1

Table 4. Indications for Esophagogastroduodenoscopy (EGD) (N=270,957), 2001–2005 (continued)

INDICATION		PERCENTAGE[1]
FOLLOWUP OF DIAGNOSIS	Positive Fecal Occult Blood Test	2.7
	Suspected Upper Gastrointestinal Bleed	2.5
	Abnormal Study/Exam/Results	2.1
	Therapeutic Intervention	1.2
	Evaluation of Suspected Varices	0.8
	Suspected Barrett's Esophagus	0.4
	Family History of Cancer	0.3
	Prior Upper Gastrointestinal Cancer	0.2
	Gastrointestinal Symptoms in Immunocompromised Host	0.1
	Personal History of Other Upper Gastrointestinal Condition	0.1
	Evaluation of Crohn's Disease	< 0.1
OTHER		8.4

[1] Indication categories are not mutually exclusive.

[2] Alarm symptoms = weight loss, vomiting, bleeding cluster.

[3] GERD = reflux symptoms, excluding dysphagia and surveillance of Barrett's esophagus.

[4] Dyspepsia/abdominal pain = dyspepsia and/or abdominal pain/bloating, excluding reflux symptoms; dysphagia; and surveillance of Barrett's esophagus.

[5] Bleeding cluster = any of the following indications: anemia, iron deficiency without anemia, melena, hematemesis, hematochezia, positive fecal occult blood test, suspected upper gastrointestinal bleed.

SOURCE: National Endoscopy Database/Clinical Outcomes Research Initiative

Table 5. Esophagogastroduodenoscopy (EGD) Findings (N=270,957), 2001–2005

FINDING	PERCENTAGE[1]
Normal Exam	41.5
Mucosal Abnormality	38.8
Hiatal Hernia	33.4
Esophageal Inflammation	17.8
Stricture/Stenosis	9.9
Barrett's Esophagus	6.7
Ulcer	6.3
Polyp	4.5
Varices	2.8
Prior Surgery	2.6
Foreign Body/Retained Food	2.1
Nodule	2.0
Anatomical Deformity	1.0
Tumor	0.9
Arteriovenous Malformation	0.9
Healed Ulcer	0.5
Other Finding	18.0

[1] Finding categories are not mutually exclusive.
SOURCE: National Endoscopy Database/Clinical Outcomes Research Initiative

Table 6. Endoscopic Retrograde Cholangiopancreatography (ERCP) Findings (N=9,333), 2001–2005

FINDING	PERCENTAGE[1]
Ductal Dilation	37.2
Normal Exam	34.6
Stones	25.9
Stricture/Stenosis	18.1
Filling Defect	8.5
Duodenal Diverticulum	5.7
Stent	4.6
Leak/Extravasation	3.1
Irregularity	2.3
Tumor	1.5
Pancreas Divisum	1.0
Pancreatitis	0.7
Extrinsic Compression	0.5
Pancreatic Pseudocyst	0.4
Cholangitis	0.3
Other Finding	28.2

[1] Finding categories are not mutually exclusive.
SOURCE: National Endoscopy Database/Clinical Outcomes Research Initiative

CHAPTER 25
Costs of Digestive Diseases

Constance E. Ruhl, M.D., Ph.D.; Bryan Sayer, M.H.S.; Danita D. Byrd-Holt, B.B.A.; and Douglas M. Brown, Ph.D.

This chapter provides the estimated costs of digestive diseases in the United States for 2004, the last year for which data were available from all sources used in this analysis. Direct medical costs included expenditures for hospital services, physician services, prescription drugs, over-the-counter drugs, nursing home care, home health care, hospice care, and outpatient endoscopy. Indirect costs of morbidity and mortality associated with digestive diseases were also calculated.

The costs of digestive diseases were estimated using the human capital approach.[1, 2] Costs under the human capital method include the value of resources used for medical care (direct costs) and those forgone due to time lost from work and leisure (indirect costs). To calculate direct costs, billed charges are used as an imperfect surrogate for the sum of all the resource payments used in the production of patient services for which data are unavailable. For hospital facilities, costs obtained from the Healthcare Cost and Utilization Project Nationwide Inpatient Sample (HCUP NIS) (Appendix 2) were converted from total charges using cost-to-charge ratios based on hospital accounting reports from the Centers for Medicare & Medicaid Services.

Where possible, an attempt was made to provide cost estimates by ICD codes for each digestive disease with a substantial economic impact. Digestive disease definitions were based on ICD-9-CM codes for health care and ICD-10 codes for mortality, as listed in Appendix 1.

The methodology used to derive cost estimates for digestive diseases is briefly described here. More detail is to be made available at a National Institutes of Health Web site (http://www2.niddk.nih.gov/). A conservative approach was taken toward estimation of economic costs. A limitation of this approach is an underestimate of indirect costs related to work loss from digestive diseases not related to medical care (discussion follows).

DIRECT COSTS

Direct costs represent charges for hospital services, physician services, prescription drugs, over-the-counter drugs, nursing home care, home health care, hospice care, and outpatient endoscopy.

Hospital facility costs and physician charges for hospital and ambulatory care include only non-Federal hospitals and physicians, and, therefore, underestimate the total costs of hospital care and ambulatory care for digestive diseases in the United States. (Federal hospitals and physicians include those of the armed services, Department of Veterans Affairs, and the Indian Health Service.) Approximately 10 percent of care in the United States is provided by non-reported hospitals and physicians.

Hospital facility costs (Table 2, column 2) were taken from the 2004 HCUP NIS, a representative sample of hospital discharges from non-Federal hospitals in the United States (Appendix 2). Some hospital facility costs were assumed to be associated with problems other than the first-listed diagnosis. Therefore, 80 percent of inpatient facility charges were allocated to the primary diagnosis (or 100 percent if no secondary diagnoses were present). The remaining 20 percent was allocated to the secondary diagnoses in proportion to the number of secondary diagnoses. For example, if there were three secondary diagnoses, each one received one-third of 20 percent of these costs. If two of the three secondary diagnoses were digestive diseases, then those two each received one-third of 20 percent of the total, and the other one-third was not included, because it was associated with a nondigestive disease.

Total hospital facility costs were $40.6 billion. Facility charges for first-listed diagnoses were 86 percent of the total hospital charges. Diseases costing more than $1 billion (in descending order) were gallstones, abdominal wall hernia, diverticular disease, pancreatitis, colorectal cancer, appendicitis, liver disease, GERD, and peptic ulcer disease.

Physician hospital charges (Table 2, column 3) include those for performing procedures and those for patient visits (rounds). Data on number of hospital discharges with a diagnosis of each digestive disease, as well as length of stay and procedures performed at those visits, were taken from the 2004 HCUP NIS. Because no national estimates were available for the average price charged by physicians per procedure, Medicare reimbursement rates were used. These rates are locality-specific; therefore, we used the average of the regional reimbursement rates weighted by the population density of each region. As in the calculation of hospital facility costs, 80 percent of physician procedure charges were allocated to the primary diagnosis and 20 percent to secondary diagnoses.

To estimate physician visit charges, Medicare reimbursement rates were used. It was assumed that for each first-listed diagnosis there was one physician visit per day in the hospital, and that when a digestive disease was a secondary diagnosis, an average of one visit per hospitalization by a second physician would have occurred for each secondary digestive disease diagnosis.

Two surgical procedures, laparoscopic cholecystectomy (ICD-9-CM procedure code 51.23) and inguinal herniorrhaphy (ICD-9-CM 53.0–53.1), are frequently performed as ambulatory surgery. For each of these procedures, the number of ambulatory surgeries was estimated as the difference between the total number of surgeries (inpatient and outpatient) in 1996, the last year for which ambulatory surgery data were available, and the number of inpatient surgeries in 2004. Facility charges were approximated as the average charge for a 1-day overnight hospitalization for the same procedure. Physician charges were estimated by Medicare reimbursement rates. The total cost of ambulatory laparoscopic cholecystectomies was estimated to be $2.0 billion, and the total cost of ambulatory herniorrhaphies was estimated to be $2.5 billion. These costs were included in hospital and physician hospital costs for gallstone disease and abdominal wall hernia, respectively, in Table 2.

Additional costs that could not be distributed among individual digestive diseases were from services provided by primarily hospital-based specialties: anesthesiology, radiology, and pathology. Their costs were estimated by multiplying the amount of collection for professional charges for each specialty by the number of physicians involved in patient care for each specialty.[3, 4] Anesthesiology costs included those for certified nurse anesthetists.[5] The cost attributable to digestive diseases was estimated as 12 percent of total costs for each specialty; 12 percent was based on the average calculation from the HCUP NIS of the proportion of all hospital discharges, all hospital facility costs, and all physician hospital costs attributed to digestive diseases.

Total physician charges associated with hospital services for digestive diseases were $14.7 billion. Procedures performed at the hospital (including anesthesiology costs) accounted for $5.5 billion and physician hospital visits for $5.2 billion (remaining costs were attributed to radiologists, pathologists, and ambulatory herniorrhaphy and cholecystectomy). Procedures performed for first-listed diagnoses were 85 percent of the total procedure charges. Visits made for first-listed diagnoses were 42 percent of the total visit charges, while consultant fees for secondary diagnoses accounted for the remainder. GERD, gallstones, and abdominal wall hernia had the highest physician fees.

Ambulatory care costs (Table 2, column 4) consist of physician fees for office visits plus any extra charges for procedures performed in their offices. Data on number of ambulatory visits with a diagnosis of each digestive disease and services provided at those visits were taken from the 2004 National Ambulatory Medical Care Survey (NAMCS) and the 2004 National Hospital Ambulatory Medical Care Survey (NHAMCS), representative samples of office-based and hospital-based, respectively, non-Federal physicians in the United States (Appendix 2). Only the primary diagnosis was used for ambulatory care estimates. Medicare reimbursement rates were used to estimate physician visit fees and procedure charges.

Total ambulatory care costs (excluding ambulatory surgery) were $16.0 billion. Procedures performed on outpatients constituted 50 percent of this amount. Abdominal wall hernia, GERD, chronic constipation, gallstones, and diverticular disease were the largest contributors to ambulatory costs.

Expenditures for prescription drugs written by physicians during an office visit (Table 2, column 5) were derived using national data for 2004 collected by Verispan (Appendix 2). They were based on first-listed diagnoses only. For some digestive diseases, numbers were too small to produce reliable estimates.

The total cost of prescription drugs was $12.3 billion. Over half of this cost ($7.7 billion) was associated with drugs prescribed for GERD. Peptic ulcer disease, hepatitis C, IBS, and IBD were major contributors to the remaining drug cost.

Nursing home costs (Table 2, column 6) were estimated using data from the 2004 National Nursing Home Survey (NNHS) (Appendix 2). Home health care costs (Table 2, column 7) and hospice care costs (Table 2, column 8) were estimated using data from the 2000 National Home and Hospice Care Survey (NHHCS) (Appendix 2). Expenditures for home health and hospice care were inflated to estimate 2004 costs. For both surveys, costs were calculated using the average daily rate and the length of stay and were allocated among primary and secondary diagnoses using an 80-20 split. For some digestive diseases, data were unavailable.

Nursing home costs totaled $3.3 billion. The conditions making the largest contributions to these costs were GERD, chronic constipation, diverticular disease, peptic ulcer disease, and colorectal cancer.

Home health care costs totaled $3.1 billion. The conditions making the largest contributions to these costs were colorectal cancer, Crohn's disease, and pancreatic cancer. Hospice care costs totaled an additional $1.9 billion, with the largest contributors to cost being colorectal, pancreatic, and gastric cancers.

Two additional categories of direct costs could not be distributed among individual digestive diseases: outpatient endoscopy and over-the-counter drugs (Table 2). Endoscopic procedures performed among

outpatients are inadequately captured by the NAMCS and the NHAMCS. To estimate costs of outpatient endoscopy, national estimates of the number of colonoscopies and flexible sigmoidoscopies (performed in 2002) were obtained from the Survey of Endoscopic Capacity (SECAP), conducted by the Centers for Disease Control and Prevention and adjusted to 2004 levels based on trends in the CORI (Appendix 2).[6] The number of EGDs was estimated using the ratio of EGDs to colonoscopies from CORI. From these totals, the numbers accounted in the outpatient and inpatient data are subtracted, leaving the total number of procedures missed by those data. Medicare reimbursement rates were used to estimate these additional endoscopy charges. Outpatient endoscopy costs were estimated to be $3.7 billion.

An estimate of expenditures for over-the-counter drugs (for GERD, constipation, and diarrhea) was obtained from retail trade data provided by the Consumer Healthcare Products Association.[7] These costs represent sales to major pharmacy markets, excluding Walmart. Adding Walmart's share, estimated to be 10 percent of sales in this market, yields an estimated total of $2.1 billion.

The total direct cost of digestive diseases in the United States in 2004 was estimated to be $97.8 billion (Table 2). Hospital facility costs and physician hospital costs accounted for 57 percent. Over $85 billion of this total could be assigned to individual digestive diseases. The remaining $12.1 billion, which could not be allocated to individual diseases, represented unassigned outlays for hospital-based physicians, outpatient endoscopy, and over-the-counter drugs. The 10 most significant digestive diseases in terms of direct costs in 2004 were (in descending order) GERD, gallstones, AWH, colorectal cancer, diverticular disease, peptic ulcer disease, pancreatitis, liver disease, appendicitis, and chronic constipation. These 10 diseases cost $42.8 billion, which represented 44 percent of total costs, or 50 percent of expenditures assigned to individual diseases. Neoplasms accounted for $8.4 billion, or 10 percent of the direct costs assigned to individual diseases.

INDIRECT COSTS

Indirect costs comprise the implicit value of forgone earnings or production due to (1) consumption of hospital or ambulatory care, (2) premature death, and (3) additional work loss associated with acute and chronic digestive diseases. Indirect costs also include the value of leisure time lost due to morbidity and mortality.

To determine forgone earnings and leisure due to hospital stays, ambulatory care visits, and death, data were obtained from the U.S. Department of Commerce, Bureau of Labor Statistics, Employment and Earnings. For each age group, the average wage paid, including benefits, and the average employment rate (as a proxy for the probability that a person would have been working) were used. For children under 15 years of age, the costs of forgone earnings and leisure due to hospitalization or physician office visits were those of adults who were assumed to have accompanied the children. In calculating indirect costs, 100 percent of costs were attributed to the first-listed diagnosis.

Indirect costs due to hospital stays (Table 3, column 2), were estimated by obtaining data from the 2004 HCUP NIS on number of days hospitalized by condition and age. For this calculation, it was assumed conservatively that patients would spend twice the equivalent number of days at home recuperating as spent in the hospital.

The total indirect cost due to hospital stays was $5.8 billion. Pancreatitis, liver disease, diverticular disease, and gallstones were the most significant causes of lost wages during hospital stays.

Indirect costs due to ambulatory visits (Table 3, column 3) were estimated in a similar manner to those for hospital stays, except for the assumption that the average visit took 1 hour and 50 minutes away from work or leisure.[8]

The total indirect cost due to ambulatory visits was $1.9 billion. The largest contributors to this cost were GERD and AWHs.

Indirect costs of lost earnings and leisure due to premature death (Table 3, column 4) were estimated using the number of deaths in 2004 and the projected future lifetime earnings, benefits, and leisure for men and women to age 75, based on age at death.[9] The expected lifetime value was discounted to the present using a 4 percent annual discount rate; 100 percent of costs were attributed to the underlying cause of death.

The total indirect cost due to mortality was $32.8 billion. Liver disease was the costliest condition at $10.2 billion. Because of their high fatality rate, digestive tract malignancies accounted for a large proportion of the mortality costs (46 percent).

A major source of indirect costs that could not be assigned to individual digestive diseases was the cost of work and leisure loss from acute and chronic conditions that did not result in a physician outpatient visit or hospitalization. An estimate of the total number of days lost was obtained from the Medical Expenditure Panel Survey (MEPS) (Appendix 2) and converted to dollars using the age- and sex-specific rates of forgone earnings. Losses captured by inpatient and outpatient encounters are subtracted from this total. The resulting indirect cost of conditions not resulting in medical care or death was estimated at $3.6 billion. In contrast, the cost estimate for work loss days in 1985 from acute gastroenteritis alone was $4.1 billion.[10] In MEPS, any acute condition that resulted in work loss was obtained by self-report of that condition, which is a concern for self-limited illnesses that do not require visits to a health care provider.

The total indirect cost of digestive diseases in the United States in 2004 was estimated at $44.0 billion (Table 2). Almost three-quarters of this cost was due to mortality, and one-fourth was from work loss due to medical care or illness. Liver disease, colorectal cancer, and pancreatic cancer resulted in the greatest indirect costs.

The total estimated cost of digestive diseases, including direct and indirect, in the United States in 2004 was $141.8 billion (Table 1). Direct costs accounted for 69 percent of the total. The majority of costs (88 percent of direct and 92 percent of indirect) was assigned to specific digestive diseases. In total cost, the most costly diseases were liver disease ($13.1 billion), GERD ($12.6 billion), colorectal cancer ($9.5 billion), gallstones ($6.2 billion), and AWH ($6.1 billion).

Our cost calculations have limitations: (1) Hospital facility costs and physician charges for hospital and ambulatory care include only non-Federal hospitals and physicians, and, therefore, underestimate the total cost of hospital care and ambulatory care for digestive diseases in the United States. (2) Physician costs for procedures were based on Medicare reimbursement rates, which may differ from (i.e., be lower than) rates of other payers. (3) Physician costs for inpatient and outpatient visits were based on Medicare reimbursement rates, which may differ from (i.e., be lower than) rates of other payers. (4) Over-the-counter drug data did not include all categories of digestive disease drugs. (5) Indirect costs of acute and chronic conditions that did not result in medical care did not include data for all digestive diseases. (6) Indirect costs do not include work loss due to disability, for which we have no data. Consequently, the true cost of digestive diseases in the United States is underestimated.

REFERENCES

1 Hodgson TA. The state of the art of cost-of-illness estimates. *Advances in health economics and health service research.* 1983;4:129-164.

2 Brown DM, Everhart JE. Cost of digestive disease in the United States. In: Everhart JE, editor. *Digestive diseases in the United States: epidemiology and impact.* US Department of Health and Human Services, Public Health Service, National Institutes of Health, National Institute of Diabetes and Digestive and Kidney Diseases. Washington, DC: US Government Printing Office, 1994; NIH Publication No. 94-1447 pp. 57–82.

3 Medical Group Management Association. *Physician compensation and production survey.* Englewood, Colorado: Center for Research in Ambulatory Health Care Administration, 2005.

4 American Medical Association (AMA). *Physician characteristics and distribution in the US*, 2006 Edition. Chicago: AMA, 2006. pp. 20–24.

5 US Government Accountability Office (GAO). *Medicare physician payments: Medicare and private payment differences for anesthesia services.* GAO-07-463, Washington, DC: July 2007.

6 Seeff LC, Richards TB, Shapiro JA, Nadel MR, Manninen DL, Given LS, Dong FB, Winges LD, McKenna MT. How many endoscopies are performed for colorectal cancer screening? Results from CDC's survey of endoscopic capacity. *Gastroenterology* 2004;127:1670-7.

7 Accessed at http://www.chpa-info.org.

8 American Medical Association (AMA). *Physician and socioeconomic statistics.* 2003 Edition. Chicago: AMA, 2003.

9 Accessed at http://data.bls.gov/cgi-bin/surveymost.

10 Brown and Everhart, op. cit.

Table 1. Direct, Indirect, and Total Costs of Digestive Diseases in the United States, 2004 ($ Millions)

DIGESTIVE DISEASE	Direct Costs	Indirect Costs	TOTAL
Gastrointestinal Infections	$1,343.4	$392.5	$1,735.9
Hepatitis A	14.5	18.5	32.9
Hepatitis B	204.6	253.2	457.9
Hepatitis C	1,065.5	1,783.6	2,849.1
Other Viral Hepatitis	15.9	32.0	47.9
All Viral Hepatitis	1,300.5	2,087.3	3,387.8
Esophageal Cancer	597.3	1,975.4	2,572.6
Gastric Cancer	487.5	1,415.0	1,902.6
Cancer of Small Intestine	123.8	159.9	283.8
Colorectal Cancer	4,043.7	5,455.2	9,498.9
Primary Liver Cancer	261.2	1,318.6	1,579.8
Bile Duct Cancer	166.0	515.5	681.5
Gallbladder Cancer	66.6	150.6	217.2
Pancreatic Cancer	1,077.4	3,225.6	4,303.0
Other Digestive Cancers	1,618.0	1,490.9	3,108.9
All Digestive Cancers	8,441.5	15,706.7	24,148.2
Hemorrhoids	775.8	97.6	873.4
Gastroesophageal Reflux Disease	12,125.0	515.0	12,639.9
Peptic Ulcer Disease	2,599.9	518.7	3,118.6
Chronic Constipation	1,572.1	140.4	1,712.5
Irritable Bowel Syndrome	949.8	57.5	1,007.3
Other Functional Intestinal Disorders	1,139.3	129.7	1,269.0
All Functional Intestinal Disorders	3,661.2	327.7	3,988.8
Appendicitis	2,310.6	356.3	2,666.8
Abdominal Wall Hernia	5,698.9	371.9	6,070.8
Crohn's Disease	1,071.0	227.9	1,298.9
Ulcerative Colitis	767.9	100.1	868.0
All Inflammatory Bowel Disease	1,838.9	328.0	2,166.9
Diverticular Disease	3,569.3	471.9	4,041.2

Table 1. Direct, Indirect, and Total Costs of Digestive Diseases in the United States, 2004 ($ Millions) (continued)

DIGESTIVE DISEASE	Direct Costs	Indirect Costs	TOTAL
Liver Disease	2,532.0	10,563.0	13,095.0
Gallstones	5,763.6	406.2	6,169.7
Pancreatitis	2,546.2	1,187.1	3,733.3
Other Digestive Diseases	31,193.0	7,102.2	38,295.2
All Digestive Diseases	85,699.7	40,432.0	126,131.7
Total Costs That Could Not Be Allocated to Specific Conditions	12,118.1	3,576.4	15,694.5
TOTAL	$97,817.9	$44,008.4	$141,826.3

Table 2. Direct Costs of Digestive Diseases in the United States, 2004 ($ Millions)

DIGESTIVE DISEASE	Hospital (Non-Federal)	Physician Hospital (Non-Federal)	Ambulatory (Non-Federal)	Prescription Drugs	Nursing Home	Home Health Care (2000)	Hospice Care (2000)	TOTAL
Gastrointestinal Infections	$877.2	$145.4	$260.0	$45.1	$9.6	$6.2	—	$1,343.4
Hepatitis A	10.9	2.6	0.9	—	0.1	0.0	—	14.5
Hepatitis B	48.3	16.8	71.8	66.7	—	0.4	0.6	204.6
Hepatitis C	206.9	95.8	241.8	506.0	—	12.7	2.3	1,065.5
Other Viral Hepatitis	8.9	1.5	3.7	—	0.6	0.9	0.4	15.9
All Viral Hepatitis	274.9	116.6	318.2	572.8	0.7	14.0	3.3	1,300.5
Esophageal Cancer	302.2	49.9	99.7	8.7	0.7	42.3	93.7	597.3
Gastric Cancer	234.8	39.0	35.1	18.4	6.0	24.4	129.8	487.5
Cancer of Small Intestine	92.8	17.2	4.2	—	—	0.0	9.7	123.8
Colorectal Cancer	1,947.4	392.4	465.5	81.0	122.4	277.5	757.5	4,043.7
Primary Liver Cancer	151.7	24.9	26.5	—	33.0	—	25.1	261.2
Bile Duct Cancer	119.1	21.3	7.1	—	—	—	18.5	166.0
Gallbladder Cancer	31.5	6.3	8.4	—	—	3.6	16.8	66.6
Pancreatic Cancer	403.7	71.0	76.3	33.3	12.4	105.9	374.8	1,077.4
Other Digestive Cancers	1,044.1	225.0	123.4	2.1	9.1	46.5	167.8	1,618.0
All Digestive Cancers	4,327.3	847.0	846.2	143.5	183.7	500.1	1,593.7	8,441.5
Hemorrhoids	196.7	79.6	447.3	43.0	7.4	1.8	—	775.8
Gastroesophageal Reflux Disease	1,527.4	774.8	1,391.1	7,689.8	641.9	82.4	17.6	12,125.0
Peptic Ulcer Disease	1,442.5	246.9	199.0	518.6	130.6	61.4	0.9	2,599.9
Chronic Constipation	297.5	154.4	627.3	178.2	254.6	59.0	1.0	1,572.1
Irritable Bowel Syndrome	113.8	50.9	467.2	294.7	19.6	3.3	0.4	949.8

Table 2. Direct Costs of Digestive Diseases in the United States, 2004 ($ Millions) (continued)

DIGESTIVE DISEASE	Hospital (Non-Federal)	Physician Hospital (Non-Federal)	Ambulatory (Non-Federal)	Prescription Drugs	Nursing Home	Home Health Care (2000)	Hospice Care (2000)	TOTAL
Other Functional Intestinal Disorders	429.6	111.8	217.7	270.6	88.6	16.3	4.7	1,139.3
All Functional Intestinal Disorders	840.9	317.0	1,312.2	743.5	362.8	78.7	6.2	3,661.2
Appendicitis	1,930.7	261.1	92.2	5.6	15.4	5.6	—	2,310.6
Abdominal Wall Hernia	3,527.6	541.9	1,496.4	59.5	22.2	49.8	1.6	5,698.9
Crohn's Disease	427.1	78.3	160.6	261.5	6.2	137.2	0.1	1,071.0
Ulcerative Colitis	296.3	58.1	113.7	272.9	6.4	20.5	0.1	767.9
All Inflammatory Bowel Disease	723.4	136.3	274.3	534.4	12.6	157.8	0.2	1,838.9
Diverticular Disease	2,239.0	421.2	553.8	100.2	181.8	71.0	2.2	3,569.3
Liver Disease	1,799.9	310.1	214.6	16.1	62.1	45.3	84.0	2,532.0
Gallstones	4,314.6	748.1	619.1	18.6	41.9	21.1	0.1	5,763.6
Pancreatitis	1,982.2	258.0	85.5	88.6	50.5	75.8	5.7	2,546.2
Other Digestive Diseases	14,630.3	3,285.8	7,875.6	1,752.6	1,552.5	1,885.6	210.6	31,193.0
All Digestive Diseases	40,634.6	8,489.8	15,985.5	12,331.7	3,275.6	3,056.6	1,925.8	85,699.7
Total Costs That Could Not Be Allocated to Specific Conditions								
Over-the-Counter Drugs								2,141.0
Outpatient Endoscopy			3,718.5					3,718.5
Hospital-Based Physicians		6,258.6						6,258.6
TOTAL								$97,817.9

Table 3. Indirect Costs of Digestive Diseases in the United States, 2004 ($ Millions)

DIGESTIVE DISEASE	Hospital Stay	Ambulatory Care	Mortality	TOTAL
Gastrointestinal Infections	$165.6	$65.8	$161.1	$392.5
Hepatitis A	2.5	0.2	15.8	18.5
Hepatitis B	10.1	15.4	227.7	253.2
Hepatitis C	46.7	51.2	1,685.7	1,783.6
Other Viral Hepatitis	2.0	1.2	28.9	32.0
All Viral Hepatitis	61.3	68.0	1,958.0	2,087.3
Esophageal Cancer	41.8	9.1	1,924.5	1,975.4
Gastric Cancer	31.5	2.3	1,381.3	1,415.0
Cancer of Small Intestine	12.1	0.3	147.5	159.9
Colorectal Cancer	226.3	38.1	5,190.8	5,455.2
Primary Liver Cancer	22.5	2.3	1,293.8	1,318.6
Bile Duct Cancer	14.1	0.7	500.6	515.5
Gallbladder Cancer	3.5	1.1	146.1	150.6
Pancreatic Cancer	54.9	7.5	3,163.2	3,225.6
Other Digestive Cancers	148.5	6.4	1,336.0	1,490.9
All Digestive Cancers	555.3	67.7	15,083.7	15,706.7
Hemorrhoids	32.9	59.8	5.0	97.6
Gastroesophageal Reflux Disease	231.6	194.8	88.5	515.0
Peptic Ulcer Disease	181.8	16.3	320.6	518.7
Chronic Constipation	52.3	75.6	12.4	140.4
Irritable Bowel Syndrome	21.8	35.4	0.4	57.5
Other Functional Intestinal Disorders	80.1	26.7	22.9	129.7
All Functional Intestinal Disorders	154.2	137.7	35.7	327.7
Appendicitis	264.1	19.6	72.5	356.3
Abdominal Wall Hernia	160.3	107.3	104.3	371.9
Crohn's Disease	84.8	25.1	118.1	227.9
Ulcerative Colitis	56.7	11.6	31.8	100.1
All Inflammatory Bowel Disease	141.5	36.6	149.9	328.0
Diverticular Disease	314.9	36.0	120.9	471.9
Liver Disease	345.2	38.2	10,179.6	10,563.0

Table 3. Indirect Costs of Digestive Diseases in the United States, 2004 ($ Millions) (continued)

DIGESTIVE DISEASE	Hospital Stay	Ambulatory Care	Mortality	TOTAL
Gallstones	303.4	32.1	70.7	406.2
Pancreatitis	398.2	13.0	775.9	1,187.1
Other Digestive Diseases	2,485.5	983.3	3,633.4	7,102.2
All Digestive Diseases	5,795.9	1,876.2	32,759.8	40,432.0
Total Costs That Could Not Be Allocated to Specific Conditions				
Additional Work Loss				3,576.4
TOTAL				$44,008.4

ICD and SEER Codes

Table 1. International Classification of Diseases (ICD) Code Disease Definitions

DISEASE CODE	DIGESTIVE DISEASE	ICD-9-CM Codes for Morbidity	ICD-9 Codes for Mortality (1979–1998)	ICD-10 Codes for Mortality (1999–2004)
1	Gastrointestinal Infections	001–009	001–009	A00–A09
2	Hepatitis A	070.0, 070.1	070.0, 070.1	B15
3	Hepatitis B	1991–PRESENT: 070.42, 070.52 ALL YEARS: 070.2, 070.3	070.2, 070.3	B16, B17.0, B18.0, B18.1
4	Hepatitis C	1991–PRESENT: 070.41, 070.44, 070.51, 070.54, 070.7 BEFORE 1991: 070.4, 070.5	070.4, 070.5	B17.1, B18.2
5	Other Viral Hepatitis	1991–PRESENT: 070.43, 070.49, 070.53, 070.59 ALL YEARS 070.6, 070.9	070.6, 070.9	B17.2, B17.8, B18.8, B18.9, B19
2–5	All Viral Hepatitis	—	—	—
6	Esophageal Cancer	150, 151.0	150, 151.0	C15, C16.0
7	Gastric Cancer	151.1–151.9	151.1–151.9	C16.1–C16.9
8	Cancer of Small Intestine	152	152	C17
9	Colorectal Cancer	153, 154.0–154.1	153, 154.0–154.1	C18–C20
10	Primary Liver Cancer	155.0	155.0	C22.0, C22.2–C22.7
11	Bile Duct Cancer	155.1, 156.1–156.9	155.1, 156.1–156.9	C22.1, C24
12	Gallbladder Cancer	156.0	156.0	C23
13	Pancreatic Cancer	157	157	C25
14	Other Digestive Cancers	154.2–154.3, 154.8, 155.2, 158, 159.0, 159.8, 159.9, 196.2, 197.4–197.8	154.2–154.3, 154.8, 155.2, 158, 159.0, 159.8, 159.9, 196.2, 197.4–197.8	C21, C22.9, C26.0, C26.8, C26.9, C45.1, C48.0–C48.8, C77.2, C78.4–C78.8

Table 1. International Classification of Diseases (ICD) Code Disease Definitions (continued)

DISEASE CODE	DIGESTIVE DISEASE	ICD-9-CM Codes for Morbidity	ICD-9 Codes for Mortality (1979–1998)	ICD-10 Codes for Mortality (1999–2004)
6–14	All Digestive Cancers	—	—	—
15	Hemorrhoids	455	455	I84
16	Gastroesophageal Reflux Disease	530.1–530.3, 530.81	530.1–530.3	K20, K21, K22.1, K22.2
17	Peptic Ulcer Disease	531–534	531–534	K25–K28
18	Chronic Constipation	564.0	564.0	K59.0
19	Irritable Bowel Syndrome	564.1	564.1	K58
20	Other Functional Disorders	536, 564.2–564.9	536, 564.2–564.9	K30, K31.0, K59.1–K59.9, K91.0, K91.1, K91.8
18–20	All Functional Disorders	—	—	—
21	Appendicitis	540–543	540–543	K35–K38
22	Abdominal Wall Hernia	550, 551.0–551.2, 551.8, 551.9, 552.0–552.2, 552.8, 552.9, 553.0–553.2, 553.8, 553.9	550, 551.0–551.2, 551.8, 551.9, 552.0–552.2, 552.8, 552.9, 553.0–553.2, 553.8, 553.9	K40–K43, K45, K46
23	Crohn's Disease	555	555	K50
24	Ulcerative Colitis	556	556	K51
23–24	All Inflammatory Bowel Diseases	—	—	—
25	Diverticular Disease	562	562	K57
26	Liver Disease	570–573	570–573	K70–K76
27	Gallstones	574	574	K80
28	Pancreatitis	577.0, 577.1	577.0, 577.1	K85, K86.0, K86.1
29	Other Digestive Diseases	014, 017.8, 021.1, 022.2, 032.83, 040.2, 060, 072.3, 072.71, 075, 086.1, 091.1, 091.62, 095.2, 095.3, 098.7, 098.86, 099.52, 099.56, 112.84, 112.85, 120–129, 130.5, 176.3, 211, 230.1–230.9, 235.2–235.5, 239.0, 251.4–251.9, 271.3, 273.4, 275.0, 275.1, 277.01, 277.03, 277.1, 277.4, 279.01, 280.8, 281.0, 286.0–286.5, 286.7, 289.2, 306.4, 307.54, 307.7, 452, 453.0, 456.0–456.2, 530.0, 530.4–530.7, 530.82–530.89, 530.9, 535,	014, 017.8, 021.1, 022.2, 040.2, 060, 072.3, 075, 086.1, 091.1, 095.2, 095.3, 098.7, 120–129, 130.5, 176.3, 211, 230.1–230.9, 235.2–235.5, 239.0, 251.4–251.9, 271.3, 273.4, 275.0, 275.1, 277.1, 277.4, 280.8, 281.0, 286.0–286.5, 286.7, 289.2, 306.4, 307.7, 452, 453.0, 456.0–456.2, 530.0, 530.4–530.9, 535, 537, 538, 551.3, 552.3, 553.3, 557, 558, 560, 565–569,	A18.3, A21.3, A22.2, A51.1, A54.6, A56.3, A60.1, A74.8, A95, B25.1, B25.2, B26.3, B27, B46.2, B57.3, B58.1, B65–B83, B94.2, D00.1, D00.2, D01, D12, D13, D19.1, D20, D37.1–D37.9, D48.3, D48.4, D50.1, D51.0, D66, D67, D68.0–D68.4, D80.2, E16.3–E16.9, E73, E74.3, E80, E83.0, E83.1, E84.1, E88.0, F50.5, F98.1, I81, I82.0, I85, I86.4, I88.0, I98.2, K22.0, K22.3–K22.9, K23, K29, K31.1–K31.9, K44,

Table 1. International Classification of Diseases (ICD) Code Disease Definitions (continued)

DISEASE CODE	DIGESTIVE DISEASE	ICD-9-CM Codes for Morbidity	ICD-9 Codes for Mortality (1979–1998)	ICD-10 Codes for Mortality (1999–2004)
29 (cont.)	Other Digestive Diseases (cont.)	537, 538, 551.3, 552.3, 553.3, 557, 558, 560, 565–569, 575, 576, 577.2, 577.8, 577.9, 578, 579, 643, 646.7, 671.8, 750.3–750.9, 751, 772.4, 773.4, 774.2–774.7, 776.0, 777, 779.3, 782.4, 787, 789.0, 789.1, 789.3–789.9, 792.1, 793.3, 793.4, 793.6, 794.8, 862.22, 862.32, 863, 864, 868.02–868.04, 868.12–868.14, 935.1, 935.2, 936–938, 947.2, 947.3, 973, 988.1, 996.82, 996.86, 996.87, 997.4, V01.0, V02.0–V02.3, V02.6, V03.0, V03.1, V04.4, V05.3, V06.0, V10.00, V10.03–V10.09, V12.7, V16.0, V18.5, V42.7, V42.83, V42.84, V44.1–V44.4, V45.3, V45.72, V45.75, V45.86, V47.3, V53.5, V55.1–V55.4, V58.75, V59.6, V73.4, V74.0, V75.5–V75.7, V76.41, V76.5, E858.4, E870.7, E879.5, E943	575, 576, 577.2, 577.8, 577.9, 578, 579, 643, 646.7, 671.8, 750.3–750.9, 751, 772.4, 773.4, 774.2–774.7, 776.0, 777, 779.3, 782.4, 787, 789.0, 789.1, 789.3–789.9, 792.1, 793.3, 793.4, 793.6, 794.8, 863, 864, 935.1, 935.2, 936–938, 947.2, 947.3, 973, 988.1, 997.4	K52, K55, K56, K60–K63, K65–K67, K81–K83, K86.2–K86.9, K87, K90, K91.2–K91.5, K91.9, K92, K93 O21, O22.4, O26.6, P53, P54.0–P54.3, P57, P59, P75–P78, P92.0, P92.1, Q39–Q45, R10.0, R10.1, R10.3, R10.4, R11–R15, R16.0, R16.2, R17–R19, R93.2, R93.3, R93.5, R94.5, S36.1–S36.9, T18.1–T18.9, T28.1, T28.2, T28.6, T28.7, T47, T62.0, T85.5, T86.4, Y53, Y60.7, Y84.5, Z11.0, Z11.6, Z12.0, Z12.1, Z20.0, Z20.5, Z22.0, Z22.1, Z22.5, Z23.0, Z23.1, Z24.3, Z24.6, Z27.0, Z43.1–Z43.4, Z46.5, Z52.6, Z80.0, Z83.7, Z85.0, Z87.1, Z90.3, Z90.4, Z93.1–Z94.4, Z98.0
1–29	All Digestive Diseases	—	—	—

SOURCE: ICD-9-CM: http://www.cdc.gov/nchs/icd9.htm
ICD-9: http://www.cdc.gov/nchs/about/major/dvs/icd9des.htm
ICD-10: http://www.cdc.gov/nchs/about/major/dvs/icd10des.htm

Table 2. Surveillance, Epidemiology, and End Results (SEER) Program Site Recodes With SEER Morphology Codes (ICD-0-3) for Digestive Cancers

DISEASE CODE	CANCER	SEER SITE RECODES (Morphology Codes in Parentheses)
1	Esophageal Cancer, Squamous Cell	21010 (805–808)
2	Esophageal Cancer, Adenocarcinoma	21010 (814–838)
3	Esophageal Cancer, Other	21010 (all other O codes)
1–3	All Esophageal Cancer	—
4	Gastric Cancer	21020
5	Cancer of Small Intestine	21030
6	Colorectal Cancer	21041–21049, 21051, 21052
7	Primary Liver Cancer	21071
8	Bile Duct Cancer	21072, 21090
9	Gallbladder Cancer	21080
10	Pancreatic Cancer	21100
11	Other Digestive Cancers (Other Ill-Defined)	21060, 21110, 21120, 21130
1–11	All Digestive Cancers	—

SOURCE: Fritz A, Percy C, Jack A, Shanmugaratnam K, Sobin L, Parkin DM, Whelan S, eds. *International Classification of Diseases for Oncology.* 3rd ed. Geneva: World Health Organization; 2000.

APPENDIX 2

Summary of Surveys Used in *The Burden of Digestive Diseases in the United States*

Constance E. Ruhl, M.D., Ph.D.; and Bryan Sayer, M.H.S.

National Ambulatory Medical Care Survey (NAMCS)

Sponsor	Ambulatory Care Statistics Branch Division of Health Care Statistics National Center for Health Statistics Centers for Disease Control and Prevention U.S. Department of Health and Human Services 3311 Toledo Road Hyattsville, MD 20782 301-458-4600 http://www.cdc.gov/nchs/about/major/ahcd/ahcd1.htm
Design	The National Ambulatory Medical Care Survey (NAMCS) is a continuing series of nationally representative sample surveys of office-based physicians in the United States. The survey includes all non-Federal office-based physicians who are primarily engaged in direct patient care. Anesthesiologists, pathologists, and radiologists are excluded. The design is a multistage stratified probability sample of geographically defined areas, physician practices within these areas, and patient visits within physician practices. Physicians are asked to complete a patient encounter form for a systematic sample of office visits occurring during a randomly assigned 1-week reporting period. The study design is described in: National Center for Health Statistics, Bryant E, Shimuzu I. *Sample design, sampling variance, and estimation procedures for the National Ambulatory Medical Care Survey.* Hyattsville, Maryland: Public Health Service, 1988; DHHS Publication No. (PHS) 88-1382. (*Vital and health statistics*, Series 2, No. 108.)
Timeframe	Data were collected annually from 1974 through 1981, and in 1985; data have been collected annually since 1989. Data from 1992 through 2005 were used in this report.
Sample Size	Through 1981, the sample included 3,000 total physicians, about 1,925 responding physicians, and about 51,000 patient visits. The 1985 sample included about 5,000 total physicians, 2,900 responding physicians, and 70,000 patient visits. Beginning in 1989, the sample included 2,500 total physicians, about 1,600 responding physicians, and about 42,000 patient visits.
Content Relevant to Digestive Diseases	Demographic data, reason for visit, physician's diagnostic and therapeutic services ordered or provided, diagnosis and disposition decision, and drugs prescribed are included. International Classification of Diseases (ICD) codes are given for the first four physician diagnoses. The reason for office visit is the principal reason given by the patient, which in the physician's judgment is the most appropriate one. Two additional symptoms or other reasons for visit can be coded.
Strengths	The survey form is completed from provider records. Trend data are available for about 30 years. Visits can be compared with those of the National Health Inteview Survey, in which the conditions are similarly defined. Since 1980, data have been collected on the number and names of specific drugs prescribed in office-based practice. The sample allows estimates for specific physician subspecialties. ICD codes are used for diagnoses.

Limitations	The sample is limited to office-based physicians, a group that has become a less inclusive source for ambulatory care. There may be more than one report per person, because the report reflects a visit rather than an individual. The sample size is small, so estimates of fewer than 200,000 are statistically unreliable. Because ambulatory care in Federal facilities is not included, ambulatory care rates based on the U.S. population are underestimates.
Availability of Data	Published data are found in the National Center for Health Statistics *Vital and health statistics*, Series 13 (http://www.cdc.gov/nchs/products/pubs/pubd/series/ser.htm#sr13) and in *Advance data* (http://www.cdc.gov/nchs/products/pubs/pubd/ad/ad.htm). Data are available for public use on the National Center for Health Statistics Web site in an easy-to-use form with input statements.

National Hospital Ambulatory Medical Care Survey (NHAMCS)

Sponsor	Ambulatory Care Statistics Branch Division of Health Care Statistics National Center for Health Statistics Centers for Disease Control and Prevention U.S. Department of Health and Human Services 3311 Toledo Road Hyattsville, MD 20782 301-458-4600 http://www.cdc.gov/nchs/about/major/ahcd/ahcd1.htm
Design	The National Hospital Ambulatory Medical Care Survey (NHAMCS) is a continuing series of nationally representative sample surveys of physicians in hospital emergency departments and outpatient departments in the United States. The survey includes all non-institutional, non-Federal, general, and short-stay hospitals with at least six beds staffed for patient use. The design is a multistage stratified probability sample of geographically defined areas, hospitals within these areas, clinics within the outpatient departments and emergency service areas within the emergency departments of these hospitals, and patient visits to these clinics and emergency service areas. Physicians are asked to complete a patient encounter form for a systematic sample of visits occurring during a randomly assigned 4-week reporting period. The study design is described in: National Center for Health Statistics, McCaig LF, McLemore T. *Plan and operation of the National Hospital Ambulatory Medical Care Survey.* Hyattsville, Maryland: Public Health Service, 1994; DHHS Publication No. (PHS) 94-1310. (*Vital and health statistics*, Series 1, No. 34.)
Timeframe	Data have been collected annually since 1992. Data from 1992 through 2005 were used in this report.
Sample Size	A fixed panel of 600 hospitals was selected for the sample. A special supplement of 66 hospitals was added in 2003 to increase reliability of emergency department estimates for rural and proprietary hospitals. In 1992, the sample included about 36,000 emergency department visits and about 35,000 outpatient department visits.
Content Relevant to Digestive Diseases	Demographic data, reason for visit, physician's diagnostic and therapeutic services ordered or provided, diagnoses and disposition decision, drugs prescribed, types of health care professionals seen, causes of injury where applicable, expected sources of payment, and characteristics of the hospital such as type of ownership are included.
Strengths	This survey complements the NAMCS, to provide more complete data on ambulatory care. The survey form is completed from provider records. Trend data are available for more than 10 years. International Classification of Diseases (ICD) codes are used for diagnoses.
Limitations	There may be more than one report per person, because the report reflects a visit rather than an individual. The sample size is small, so estimates of fewer than 200,000 are statistically unreliable. Because ambulatory care in Federal facilities is not included, ambulatory care rates based on the U.S. population are underestimates.
Availability of Data	Published data are found in the National Center for Health Statistics *Vital and health statistics*, Series 13 (http://www.cdc.gov/nchs/products/pubs/pubd/series/ser.htm#sr13) and in *Advance data* (http://www.cdc.gov/nchs/products/pubs/pubd/ad/ad.htm). Data are available for public use on the National Center for Health Statistics Web site in an easy-to-use form with input statements.

Healthcare Cost and Utilization Project Nationwide Inpatient Sample (HCUP NIS)

Sponsor	Agency for Healthcare Research and Quality U.S. Department of Health and Human Services 540 Gaither Road, Suite 2000 Rockville, MD 20850 301-427-1364 866-290-HCUP http://www.hcup-us.ahrq.gov/
Design	The Healthcare Cost and Utilization Project Nationwide Inpatient Sample (HCUP NIS) is a database of hospital inpatient stays. It utilizes a stratified sample of hospitals drawn from the subset of hospitals in the States that make their data available to HCUP. Hospitals are stratified by region, location/teaching status, bed-size category, and ownership. All discharges from sampled hospitals are included. The 2004 HCUP NIS includes all discharges from more than 1,000 hospitals, an approximate 20 percent stratified sample of U.S. community hospitals. HCUP NIS data are weighted to represent the annual discharges from non-Federal hospitals in the United States. Several revisions have been made to the HCUP NIS sampling design since its inception. First, the sampling frame changed over time as more States made their data available to HCUP. The 1988 HCUP NIS was drawn from a sampling frame of eight States, representing 31 percent of all hospital discharges in the United States. In contrast, the sampling frame in recent years included 37 States, representing 85 to 90 percent of all hospital discharges in the United States. Second, in 1998, the sampling method was changed to better reflect the cross-sectional population of hospitals. The hospital stratification variables were redefined, short-term rehabilitation facilities were dropped from the target universe, and sampling preference was no longer given to prior-year NIS hospitals.
Timeframe	Data have been collected annually since 1988. Data from 2004 were used in this report.
Sample Size	The sample size is approximately 8 million hospital stays each year.
Content Relevant to Digestive Diseases	Data for each hospital stay include patient demographics (gender, age, race, median income for ZIP Code), admission and discharge status, length of stay, total charges, expected payment source, up to 15 diagnoses and 7 surgical procedures coded using International Classification of Diseases (ICD)-9-CM codes, and hospital characteristics (ownership, size, teaching status).
Strengths	The HCUP NIS is the largest all-payer inpatient care database in the United States. Data are weighted to be nationally representative of non-Federal hospitals in the United States. The HCUP NIS is the only national hospital database containing charge information on all patients, regardless of payer.
Limitations	Not all States participate. Not all participating States collect data on race-ethnicity; in 2004, race-ethnicity data were not collected by 11 participating States: Georgia, Illinois, Kentucky, Maine, Minnesota, Nebraska, Nevada, Ohio, Oregon, Washington, and West Virginia. The charge information is for the facility only; no information on physician fees is available. Data on medications are not supplied, although medication costs are included in the charge total.
Availability of Data	Summary statistics are published by the Agency for Healthcare Research and Quality (http://www.hcup-us.ahrq.gov/reports.jsp). An online database, HCUP-Net, allows users to generate certain statistics easily (http://hcupnet.ahrq.gov/). Selected data sets can be purchased for analysis.

National Hospital Discharge Survey (NHDS)

Sponsor	Hospital Care Statistics Branch Division of Health Care Statistics National Center for Health Statistics Centers for Disease Control and Prevention U.S. Department of Health and Human Services 3311 Toledo Road Hyattsville, MD 20782 301-458-4321 http://www.cdc.gov/nchs/about/major/hdasd/nhds.htm
Design	The National Hospital Discharge Survey (NHDS) is a continuing series of nationally representative sample surveys of hospitals in the United States. The survey includes all short-stay, non-Federal non-institutional hospitals having six or more beds for patient use and, before 1988, those in which the average length of stay for all patients was less than 30 days. In 1988, the scope was altered slightly to include all general and children's general hospitals regardless of the length of stay. The design is a two-stage stratified probability sample of hospitals and discharges within hospitals. Beginning in 1985, two data collection procedures have been used: (1) a manual system in which data are abstracted from hospital records by the hospital staff or U.S. Census Bureau staff on behalf of the National Center for Health Statistics, and (2) an automated system in which machine-readable medical record data are purchased from commercial organizations, State data systems, hospitals, or hospital associations. The study design is described in: National Center for Health Statistics, Dennison CF, Pokras R. *Design and operation of the National Hospital Discharge Survey: 1988 redesign*. Washington, D.C.: U.S. Government Printing Office, 2000; DHHS Publication No. (PHS) 2001-1315. (*Vital and health statistics*, Series 1, No. 39.)
Timeframe	Data have been collected annually since 1965. Data from 1979 through 2004 were used in this report.
Sample Size	Approximately 270,000 stays from about 500 hospitals each year constitute the sample.
Content Relevant to Digestive Diseases	Data in medical records for hospital discharges are collected for patient demographics (age, sex, race, ethnicity, and marital status), disposition, length of stay, expected source of payment, and for up to seven diagnoses and four surgical procedures coded to the International Classification of Diseases (ICD)-9-CM.
Strengths	The NHDS includes patients who die in the hospital and admissions from nursing homes, thereby producing more accurate estimates of utilization, diagnostic, and procedure data than those produced by household, self-reported interview surveys such as the National Health Interview Survey. Data are obtained directly from hospital records, thus minimizing underreporting. Data include up to seven discharge diagnoses and four procedure codes. ICD codes are used for diagnoses. Trend data are available for about 40 years.
Limitations	The data, which are based only on the factsheet of the hospital discharge record, may contain incomplete or inaccurate information, because there is no validation of condition. Extensive demographic and other health-related information is not available from hospital records. Recorded data reflect a discharge, not a person, so there may be more than one discharge per person for the same condition. Race is not coded on approximately 10 percent of records. Because hospitalizations in Federal facilities are not included, hospitalization rates based on the U.S. population are underestimates.
Availability of Data	Published data are found in the National Center for Health Statistics *Vital and health statistics*, Series 13 (http://www.cdc.gov/nchs/products/pubs/pubd/series/ser.htm#sr13) and in *Advance data* (http://www.cdc.gov/nchs/products/pubs/pubd/ad/ad.htm). Data are available for public use on data tapes, data diskettes, CD-ROMs and downloadable files from the National Center for Health Statistics Web site in an easy-to-use form with input statements.

Vital Statistics of the United States: Multiple Cause-of-Death Data

Sponsor	Mortality Statistics Branch Division of Vital Statistics National Center for Health Statistics Centers for Disease Control and Prevention U.S. Department of Health and Human Services 3311 Toledo Road, 7th floor Hyattsville, MD 20782 301-458-4666 http://www.cdc.gov/nchs/deaths.htm
Design	Multiple cause-of-death mortality data from the National Vital Statistics System provide mortality data by multiple cause of death for all deaths occurring within the United States. Each record in the microdata is based on information abstracted from death certificates filed in vital statistics offices of each State and the District of Columbia. Causes of death were coded according to the International Classification of Diseases (ICD)-9 for 1979 through 1998, and according to ICD-10, beginning in 1999. The study design is described in: National Center for Health Statistics, *Data systems of the National Center for Health Statistics*. Hyattsville, Maryland: Public Health Service, 1981; DHHS Publication No. (PHS) 82-1318. (*Vital and health statistics*: Series 1, No. 16.)
Timeframe	Data have been collected annually since 1968. Data from 1979 through 2004 were used in this report.
Sample Size	The sample is a 100 percent count of deaths in the United States.
Content Relevant to Digestive Diseases	Demographic data (age, sex, race, residence) and underlying and contributing causes of death are included.
Strengths	A complete count of deaths in the United States is included, along with 18 diagnoses. Trend data are available for more than 35 years. For digestive diseases with high mortality rates, such as cirrhosis, death records are the most comprehensive data source. Mortality statistics may be the only reliable data source for uncommon fatal conditions. Annual age-adjusted mortality rates are useful for examining trends over time, assuming case-fatality rates do not change significantly. Mortality rates for diseases that are usually fatal are often used as estimates of incidence rates when the latter are not available.
Limitations	Quality is dependent on the accuracy of death certificates, which may vary, according to condition. Chronic diseases that contribute to mortality are frequently underreported.
Availability of Data	Published data are found in: National Center for Health Statistics. *Vital statistics of the United States*, Vol. II, Mortality, Parts A and B (http://www.cdc.gov/nchs/products/pubs/pubd/vsus/vsus.htm); *National vital statistics reports* (http://www.cdc.gov/nchs/products/pubs/pubd/nvsr/nvsr.htm); and *Vital and health statistics*, Series 20 (http://www.cdc.gov/nchs/products/pubs/pubd/series/ser.htm#sr20). Data are available for public use on the National Bureau of Economic Research Web site (http://www.nber.org/data/multicause.html) in an easy-to-use form with input statements.

United States Population Estimates

Sponsor	Division of Population Projections U.S. Census Bureau From CDC Wonder Centers for Disease Control and Prevention (CDC) U.S. Department of Health and Human Services 1600 Clifton Road Atlanta, GA 30333 404-639-3311 404-639-3534 and 800-311-3435 (public inquiries) http://wonder.cdc.gov/census.html
Design	The population estimates are mid-year (July 1) population counts by age, sex, and race. The counts are used with all national samples as the denominator for all estimates of rates. The year 2000 estimates are also used for age adjusting. These estimates are not used for cancer statistics from the Surveillance, Epidemiology, and End Results (SEER) program, which has its own population counts.
Timeframe	Estimates for 1979 through 2005 were used in this report.
Sample Size	The U.S. population is the sample.
Content Relevant to Digestive Diseases	Denominators are provided for calculating rate per 100,000 persons by age, race, and sex.

Surveillance, Epidemiology, and End Results (SEER) Program

Sponsor	Cancer Statistics Branch Surveillance Research Program Division of Cancer Control and Population Sciences National Cancer Institute National Institutes of Health U.S. Department of Health and Human Services 6116 Executive Boulevard Suite 504, MSC 8316 Bethesda, MD 20892-8316 301-496-8510 http://seer.cancer.gov/
Design	A total of 17 population-based registries in the United States provide data on all residents diagnosed with cancer and follow-up information on all previously diagnosed patients. Data are compiled twice a year. Cancer mortality data are obtained from vital statistics for the entire United States.
Timeframe	Data have been collected annually since 1975. Data from 1979 through 2004 were used in this report.
Sample Size	Surveillance, Epidemiology, and End Results (SEER) program data for trends are 100 percent counts from Atlanta, Georgia; Connecticut; Detroit, Michigan; Hawaii; Iowa; New Mexico; San Francisco/Oakland, California; Seattle/Puget Sound, Washington; and Utah. SEER data for 2004 are 100 percent counts from the 9 registries above, plus Los Angeles, California; San Jose-Monterey, California; Rural Georgia; the Alaska Native Tumor Registry; Greater California; Kentucky; Louisiana; and New Jersey. National Center for Health Statistics mortality data are 100 percent counts from the entire United States.
Content Relevant to Digestive Diseases	Data regarding cancer incidence and mortality, including current and projected trends, are collected for selected sites, such as esophagus, stomach, colon, rectum, liver, and pancreas. Demographic data include age, sex, and race.
Strengths	SEER data are verified for quality and completeness. Data are estimated to be 99 percent complete from the registry sites. Mortality data are 100 percent counts of the United States. Trend data are available for about 30 years.
Limitations	SEER data represent only 17 areas of the country (and only 9 for trend data). Although the data are weighted to provide national estimates, these data are not statistically representative of the United States. Accuracy of cause of death coding for some gastrointestinal cancers is unknown.
Availability of Data	Data are published by the National Cancer Institute (http://seer.cancer.gov/publications/). Certain statistics can easily be generated online (http://seer.cancer.gov/statistics/). Selected data sets are available for analysis.

Verispan

Sponsor	Verispan 800 Township Line Road, Suite 125 Yardley, PA 19067 267-685-4300 (telephone) 267-685-4400 (fax) http://www.verispan.com/
Design	The Vector One®: National (VONA) is a national-level prescription and patient tracking service that provides data on the numbers of prescription drugs dispensed by retail pharmacies. Data on nearly half of retail prescriptions dispensed in the United States are collected each month and are projected to be nationally representative through methods that stratify by geography, pay type, and class of trade. The Physician Drug & Diagnosis Audit (PDDA) collects national-level disease state and associated therapy data from more than 3,100 office-based physicians representing 29 specialties. Physicians report all patient activity during one typical workday each month. Data collected are projected by region and specialty to be nationally representative of office-based physicians. Diagnosis data from the PDDA and prescription data from the VONA are utilized by the Factor Processor to segment the number of prescriptions, units dispensed, or retail sales by disease state or diagnosis, to estimate total number of prescriptions and total costs for specific diseases.
Timeframe	The PDDA was established in 1990. Data from 2004 were used in this report.
Sample Size	Each month, data are captured on approximately half of all retail prescriptions dispensed in the United States. More than 3,100 office-based physicians report all patient activity during 1 typical workday each month.
Content Relevant to Digestive Diseases	The database includes International Classification of Diseases (ICD) codes for physician diagnoses that can be used to generate data on drugs prescribed for specific digestive diseases of interest.
Strengths	Data are nationally representative. Drug data are available for specific diseases defined by ICD codes.
Limitations	Estimates of total numbers of prescriptions and total costs for specific diseases are based on a factoring method applying information on physician prescribing practices to pharmacy data, rather than direct measurement. Number of prescriptions written by physicians may not be equivalent to number of prescriptions filled. Retail value of drugs may not be equivalent to the cost actually paid by patients. Prescription drugs from mail-order pharmacies are not included. Over-the-counter medications are not included.
Availability of Data	Summary statistics can be purchased through a contract with Verispan.

National Endoscopy Database (NED)/Clinical Outcomes Research Initiative (CORI)

Sponsor	Clinical Outcomes Research Initiative 3303 Southwest Bond Avenue, Suite 15C Portland, OR 97239 888-786-2674 (toll-free telephone) 503-494-7401 (local telephone) 503 494-2699 (fax) 503-494-6522 (research services fax) http://www.cori.org/index.asp
Design	U.S. endoscopy sites that voluntarily participate in the Clinical Outcomes Research Initiative (CORI) submit data on all endoscopic procedures performed at the sites.
Timeframe	CORI began in 1995 and is ongoing. Data from 2001 through 2005 were used in this report.
Sample Size	Currently, more than 275,000 procedure reports are received annually from 86 practice sites and more than 400 physicians in the United States. More than 1.7 million reports exist in the National Endoscopic Database (NED). Data used in this report came from 77 practices with 101 sites that performed a total of 542,650 colonoscopies, 270,957 esophagogastroduodenoscopies (EGD), 55,708 flexible sigmoidoscopies, 9,333 endoscopic retrograde cholangiopancreatographies (ERCP), and 6,945 endoscopic ultrasonographies (EUS), from 2001 through 2005.
Content Relevant to Digestive Diseases	Data collected include site and patient characteristics, indications for procedures, findings from procedures, completion rates, and unplanned event rates.
Strengths	The NED is the only U.S. national endoscopy database. Trends can be studied using data from a subset of "stable sites" that have participated for multiple consecutive years.
Limitations	Participation in CORI is voluntary; therefore, data from participating sites are not nationally representative.
Availability of Data	Through a contract with CORI, summary statistics can be purchased by persons outside the participating endoscopy sites.

National Nursing Home Survey (NNHS)

Sponsor	Long-Term Care Statistics Branch Division of Health Care Statistics National Center for Health Statistics Centers for Disease Control and Prevention U.S. Department of Health and Human Services 3311 Toledo Road Hyattsville, MD 20782 301-458-4747 http://www.cdc.gov/nchs/nnhs.htm
Design	The National Nursing Home Survey (NNHS) is a continuing series of nationally representative sample surveys of nursing homes in the United States. The survey includes all nursing homes with at least three beds that are either certified (by Medicare or Medicaid) or have a State license to operate as a nursing home. The design is a two-stage stratified probability sample of nursing homes and of current residents, persons discharged (deceased or alive) in the past year, and staff members within nursing homes. Data on residents and discharges are collected by interviewing a nurse who obtains the needed information from the medical records and the next of kin. The redesigned 2004 survey was administered using a computer-assisted personal interviewing (CAPI) system. The study design is described in: Shimizu I. The 1985 National Nursing Home Survey design. *Proceedings of the section on survey research methods, 1986 Annual Meeting of the American Statistical Association.* Chicago: American Statistical Association, 1987.
Timeframe	Data have been collected in 1973–74, 1977, 1985, 1995, 1997, 1999, and 2004. Data from 2004 were used in this report.
Sample Size	In 2004, 1,500 facilities were selected from a sampling frame of 16,628 nursing homes, and 1,174 facilities participated. A total of 14,017 residents were sampled from the responding facilities, and 13,507 participated.
Content Relevant to Digestive Diseases	Prevalence of chronic conditions by primary diagnosis, medications taken, functional status, receipt of services (medical, nursing, and therapeutic), discharge health status and length of stay by diagnosis, cost of providing care by diagnosed condition, and sources of payment are available. Information on fecal incontinence is specifically gathered. Also included are demographic characteristics of residents, health and functional status before nursing home admission, lifetime use of nursing home care, and amount of Medicaid spending. Ostomy patients and patients with alcohol abuse or dependence can be identified. Bowel and bladder incontinence was also recorded.
Strengths	The survey provides a source of health status data on the subgroup of the population residing in and discharged from all types of nursing homes for whom health care data are otherwise difficult to obtain. Primary and secondary diagnoses by International Classification of Diseases (ICD) code, which include the diseases of the digestive system, are available for residents at admission and discharge. Reasons for admissions from short-stay hospitals by selected diagnostic-related groups for age 70 years or older include esophagitis, gastroenteritis and miscellaneous digestive disorders, and gastrointestinal hemorrhage.
Limitations	Residents with a primary diagnosis of digestive disease make up a small percentage of the nursing home population. The survey is of limited use for examining specific conditions, which tend to be coded only broadly.
Availability of Data	Published data are found in the National Center for Health Statistics *Vital and Health Statistics*, Series 13 (http://www.cdc.gov/nchs/products/pubs/pubd/series/ser.htm#sr13) and in *Advance data* (http://www.cdc.gov/nchs/products/pubs/pubd/ad/ad.htm). Data are available for public use on the National Center for Health Statistics Web site in an easy-to-use form with input statements.

National Home and Hospice Care Survey (NHHCS)

Sponsor	Long-Term Care Statistics Branch Division of Health Care Statistics National Center for Health Statistics Centers for Disease Control and Prevention U.S. Department of Health and Human Services 3311 Toledo Road Hyattsville, MD 20782 301-458-4747 http://www.cdc.gov/nchs/nhhcs.htm
Design	The National Home and Hospice Care Survey (NHHCS) is a continuing series of surveys of home and hospice care agencies in the United States. The survey includes all agencies that are licensed or certified (Medicare or Medicaid). The design is a two-stage stratified probability sample of home health and hospice agencies and of current patients and discharges within agencies. Data are collected through personal interviews with administrators and staff. The study design is described in: National Center for Health Statistics, Haupt BJ. *Development of the National Home and Hospice Care Survey.* Hyattsville, Maryland: Public Health Service, 1994; DHHS Publication No. (PHS) 94-1309. (*Vital and health statistics*, Series 1, No. 33.)
Timeframe	Data were collected in 1992, 1994, 1996, 1998, and 2000. Data from 2000 were used in this report.
Sample Size	In 2000, 1,800 agencies were selected from a sampling frame of 15,451 home health and hospice care agencies, and 1,425 agencies participated. The patient sample consisted of approximately 14,000 total patients, split between home health and hospice, and between current patients and discharged patients.
Content Relevant to Digestive Diseases	Admission and discharge diagnoses, referral and length of service, number of visits, patient charges, health status, reason for discharge, and types of services were provided.
Strengths	This survey provides a source of health status data on the subgroup of the population receiving care from, or discharged from, all types of home and hospice care agencies for whom health care data are otherwise difficult to obtain. Primary and secondary diagnoses by International Classification of Diseases (ICD) code, which include the diseases of the digestive system, are available for residents at admission and discharge.
Limitations	The exact coverage of the current patients is unclear. The weighted total may underestimate or overestimate the number of patients enrolled in a given year due to the rolling nature of the survey and the length of stay of patients. In addition, cost data represent billed amounts and not paid amounts.
Availability of Data	Published data are found in the National Center for Health Statistics *Vital and health statistics*, Series 13 (http://www.cdc.gov/nchs/products/pubs/pubd/series/ser.htm#sr13) and in *Advance data* (http://www.cdc.gov/nchs/products/pubs/pubd/ad/ad.htm). Data are available for public use on the National Center for Health Statistics Web site in an easy-to-use form with input statements.

Medical Expenditure Panel Survey (MEPS)

Sponsor	Agency for Healthcare Research and Quality U.S. Department of Health and Human Services 540 Gaither Road, Suite 2000 Rockville, MD 20850 301-427-1364 http://www.meps.ahrq.gov/mepsweb/
Design	The Medical Expenditure Panel Survey (MEPS) is a set of national surveys. The Household Component (HC) provides data from individual households and their members, which are supplemented by data from their medical providers. The HC collects data from a nationally representative subsample of households that participated in the prior year's National Health Interview Survey (NHIS). The selected subsample undergoes several rounds of interviews during 2 full years of follow-up. A new sample of households is included in the survey each year. The Medical Provider Component (MPC) surveys hospitals, physicians, home health care providers, and pharmacies identified by HC respondents to supplement and/or replace information received from the HC respondents. The Insurance Component (IC), also known as the Health Insurance Cost Study, is a separate survey of a sample of private and public sector employers that collects data on employer-based health insurance plans.
Timeframe	Data have been collected annually since 1996. Data from 2004 were used in this report.
Sample Size	The 2004 HC surveyed 32,737 individuals from 13,018 families.
Content Relevant to DIgestive Diseases	Data collected in the HC on each person in the household include demographic characteristics, health conditions, health status, use of medical services, charges and source of payments, access to care, satisfaction with care, health insurance coverage, income, and employment. Data collected in the IC include the number and types of private insurance plans offered (if any), premiums, contributions by employers and employees, eligibility requirements, benefits associated with these plans, and employer characteristics. Data utilized in the current report were from the HC and consisted of counts of the number of days of work missed due to illness, injury, or hospitalization.
Strengths	The sample is nationally representative of the U.S. population. Household data are supplemented by health care provider data. The survey includes data on number of days of work missed due to illness, injury, or hospitalization, which are unavailable from other data sources.
Limitations	Household data on medical conditions are by self-report.
Availability of Data	Summary data tables are published by the Agency for Healthcare Research and Quality on the MEPS Web site. An online database, MEPSnet, allows users to generate certain statistics easily (http://www.meps.ahrq.gov/mepsweb/data_stats/meps_query.jsp). HC data files are available for public use. IC data files are not released publicly. MPC data files are not available for public release; information from these files is incorporated into the HC data files.

APPENDIX 3
Methodology for Tables and Figures

Bryan Sayer, M.H.S.

This appendix provides information on the sources and computations for the tables and figures used in the chapters on digestive diseases.

I. DATA SOURCES

The number of ambulatory care visits, hospital discharges, and deaths in the tables and figures came from four sources (see Appendix 2 for descriptions):

1. Ambulatory care visits data in tables and figures came from the combined National Ambulatory Medical Care Survey (NAMCS)/National Hospital Ambulatory Medical Care Survey (NHAMCS) years 1992–2005 (http://www.cdc.gov/nchs/about/major/ahcd/ahcd1.htm).

2. Data on hospital discharges in the figures came from the National Hospital Discharge Survey (NHDS), years 1979–2004 (http://www.cdc.gov/nchs/about/major/hdasd/nhds.htm).

3. Hospital data in the tables came from the Healthcare Cost and Utilization Project Nationwide Inpatient Sample (HCUP NIS) for the year 2004 (http://www.hcup-us.ahrq.gov/nisoverview.jsp).

4. Mortality data came from the National Vital Statistics System Multiple Cause Mortality data years 1979–2004, as prepared by the National Bureau of Economic Research (http://www.nber.org/data/multicause.html).

For digestive cancers (Chapters 4–12), cancer incidence and survival were derived from the Surveillance, Epidemiology, and End Results (SEER) program of the National Cancer Institute (NCI) (http://seer.cancer.gov/data). Data in the tables for 2004 came from the 17 registry sites that SEER used at that time. Data in the figures for 1979–2004 were from the nine sites in operation during the entire period. Population data corresponding to the definition of the SEER sites were provided by SEER.

II. DISEASE DEFINITIONS

Digestive diseases were coded into 1 of 29 digestive disease categories based on the International Classification of Diseases (ICD)-9 CM (Clinical Modification) (http://www.cdc.gov/nchs/icd9.htm) code for morbidity, and either ICD-9 (1979–1998) or ICD-10 (1999–2004) for mortality. See Appendix 1 for the complete list of codes for each of the 29 diseases. The first-listed diagnosis was considered the primary diagnosis for tables and figures for primary digestive disease. All remaining diagnoses were considered secondary and were included under the category "All-Listed Diagnoses." In the tables and figures for ambulatory care visits, hospital discharges, and mortality, diagnoses were counted only once under the all-listed category, irrespective of the number of actual diagnoses. For example, in the chapter on all digestive diseases, only one digestive disease diagnosis was counted, even though more than one could have been listed on a medical record or death certificate.

While the coding for digestive disease mortality is generally consistent between ICD-9 and ICD-10, the World Health Organization (WHO), which produces the ICD code definitions, advises that series are not necessarily comparable across versions of the ICD code book. This change was portrayed as a vertical line at 1999 on the mortality figures.

III. DEMOGRAPHIC CATEGORIES

For the purpose of calculating rates for the U.S. population, population data were derived from the national population estimates program of the U.S. Census Bureau and the Centers for Disease Control and Prevention (CDC) (http://wonder.cdc.gov/population.html). Population counts were specific for each of the demographic subgroups shown in the tables.

DEMOGRAPHIC SUBGROUP		POPULATION COUNT, 2004
AGE (Years)	Under 15	60,806,159
	15–44	125,824,714
	45–64	70,692,944
	65+	36,333,025
RACE	White	238,285,011
	Black	38,608,953
SEX	Female	149,121,439
	Male	144,535,403
TOTAL		293,656,842

Race was coded as "White" or "Black"; or "Other," if another category was specified. Missing race data were not considered "Other." The HCUP NIS data combine Hispanic origin with race, so it was impossible to know whether Hispanics were white or black. In order not to undercount the totals, we assumed all Hispanics were white. As a result, discharges for whites were slightly overstated and for blacks slightly understated.

HCUP NIS data came from the individual States, and 11 States did not report race in 2004. To adjust for this limitation, we created a separate weight for race, based on the existing weight times the inverse of the proportion of each race in the States that did report race to the total for the United States. Note that these are counts of persons, based on the 2004 mid-year population estimate, and not the proportion of discharges. We did not report separate counts for "Other" race, because the definition in the HCUP NIS and the population counts may not be the same.

IV. AGE-ADJUSTMENT

Age-adjustment through direct standardization allowed for comparisons across race, sex, and time that were not influenced by differences in age distribution for the groups being compared. Year-specific population data in 19 age groups, plus the National Center for Health Statistics (NCHS) standard year 2000 population, were used for age-adjusting. (http://www.cdc.gov/nchs/data/nvsr/nvsr47/nvs47_03.pdf). Age-specific rates were calculated for each of the 19 age groups (age 0, age 1–4, 5-year age groups through age 84, and age 85 and older), and the results were multiplied by the year 2000 standard population proportion in each of the age groups. These results then were summed to arrive at the age-adjusted population rate estimate. Further details can be found in Anderson and Rosenberg.[1]

V. TABLES
MORBIDITY ESTIMATES

1. Ambulatory Care Visits Estimates in the tables for ambulatory care visits in 2004 were from combined NAMCS/NHAMCS files for the years 2003–2005. Multiple years were combined in order to have sufficient observations to meet the minimum threshold for reporting and for more stable estimates. The 3 years of data were averaged by dividing the sampling weight by 3, in accordance with the general instructions from NCHS. The combined file included visits to freestanding physician offices and physician offices at hospitals, and emergency room visits that did not result in an overnight stay in the hospital.

First-Listed Diagnosis The primary diagnosis for an outpatient visit was the first diagnosis listed in the record. A visit was considered to have been for 1 of the 29 digestive diseases if the first of the diagnoses listed on the record fell into the subject category. Estimates for first-listed diagnosis for digestive diseases included the number of visits and the rate of visits per 100,000 of the population. The rate per 100,000 was the number of visits, not the number of individuals with a visit, divided by the number of persons (in 100,000s) in the population in the specific subgroup.

The weighted count of visits with a first-listed diagnosis of each of the digestive diseases was the count (in thousands) listed in the table under "Ambulatory Care Visits," "First-Listed Diagnosis," "Number in Thousands." The "Rate per 100,000" was calculated by dividing the count of visits by the number of persons (in 100,000s) in the population in the specific subgroup.

All-Listed Diagnoses Each outpatient record could have multiple diagnoses listed. A visit was considered to have been for a specific digestive disease if any of the diagnoses listed on the record fell into the subject category. Therefore, any individual record could be counted for more than one digestive disease. However, a given record was not counted more than once for a specific disease. For example, a record having the ICD-9-CM diagnostic codes of "001" and "002" was only counted once in the category of Gastrointestinal Infections. The weighted count of visits with all-listed diagnoses of each of the digestive diseases was the count (in thousands) listed in the table under "Ambulatory Care Visits," "All-Listed Diagnoses," "Number in Thousands." The "Rate per 100,000" was calculated by dividing the count of visits by the number of persons in the population (in 100,000s) in the demographic subgroup.

2. Hospital Discharges Hospital discharges were based on inpatient stays of at least 1 night. Emergency room visits that did not result in an admission to the hospital with an overnight stay were not counted. Data in the tables came from the 2004 HCUP NIS file of hospital discharges from participating States. Sampling weights inflated the discharges to the U.S. total, based on information from the American Hospital Association. Data in the figures showing age-adjusted hospital discharges over time were based on the NHDS, 1979–2004.

First-Listed Diagnosis The primary diagnosis for a hospital discharge was the first diagnosis listed in the record. Inpatient estimates for first-listed diagnosis for digestive diseases included the number of discharges and the rate of discharges per 100,000 of the population. The weighted count of hospital discharges with a primary diagnosis of each of the digestive diseases was the count (in thousands) listed in the table under "Hospital Discharges," "First-Listed Diagnosis," "Number in Thousands." The "Rate per 100,000" was the number of discharges, not the number of individuals

with an inpatient stay, divided by the number of persons (in 100,000s) in the population in the specific subgroup.

All-Listed Diagnoses Each hospital discharge record could have multiple diagnoses listed. A discharge was considered to have been for a specific digestive disease if any of the diagnoses listed on the record fell into the subject category. Therefore, any individual record could be counted for more than one digestive disease. As with ambulatory care visits, a given record was not counted more than once for a specific disease. For example, ICD-9-CM diagnostic codes of "001" and "002" were only counted once in the category of Gastrointestinal Infections. The weighted count of hospital discharges with all-listed diagnoses of each of the digestive diseases was the count (in thousands) listed in the table under "Hospital Discharges," "All-Listed Diagnoses," "Number in Thousands." The "Rate per 100,000" was calculated by dividing the count of hospital discharges by the number of persons in the population (in 100,000s) in the demographic subgroup.

MORTALITY

Counts for 2004 for deaths from digestive disease were derived from the Multiple Cause-of-Death data files from the Division of Vital Statistics, CDC. These data are a complete accounting of all deaths in the United States (although not necessarily for all U.S. citizens). Cause of death is organized on a record axis, with a specific underlying cause of death and contributing causes for each decedent.

1. Underlying Cause of Death The underlying cause of death was determined from the list of all causes on the death certificate by professional coders. Underlying cause is analogous to a first-listed diagnosis for morbidity. The "Number of Deaths" column for "Underlying Cause" was a count of the number of records in the file with each digestive disease as the underlying cause of death.

The "Rate per 100,000" column was determined by dividing the number of deaths with the underlying cause by the population (in 100,000s) in the demographic subgroup. The race- and sex-specific estimates were age-adjusted, while the age-specific rates and the total were not age-adjusted.

"Years of Potential Life Lost" assumed life expectancy of 75 years, had individuals not died before that age. Because age at death is reported in full years, we added 0.5 years to each age at death. Thus, for the purpose of calculating years of life lost, a person whose age at death was listed as 65 was counted as having been 65.5 years old. The age 65.5 represented the average age of all persons who died at age 65, and each contributed 9.5 years of potential life lost (75-65.5 = 9.5). The tables showed the total number of years of life lost to age 75 in thousands.

2. Underlying or Other Cause of Death The record axis of the death certificate can contain up to 20 contributing causes in addition to the underlying cause. A recording of any of the 29 unique digestive diseases was noted for each of the 21 total possible causes, and any duplicate digestive diseases were eliminated. A death was attributed to one of the digestive diseases if any of the unduplicated digestive diseases were recorded. Therefore, a death could appear under more than one of the digestive diseases in the "Underlying or Other Cause" column of the tables. Unlike the underlying cause, only the "Number of Deaths" and the "Rate per 100,000" were shown for "Underlying or Other Cause." "Years of Potential Life Lost" were irrelevant.

"Number of Deaths" (in 100,000s) was the count of all deaths that had the specified digestive disease listed in any position on the record axis. A death could appear under more than one disease if any of the diagnoses were listed; however, no death appeared more than once for a given disease.

The "Rate per 100,000" column was determined by dividing the number of deaths for underlying or other cause by the population (in 100,000s) in the demographic subgroup. The race- and sex-specific estimates were age-adjusted, while the age-specific rates and the total were not age-adjusted.

CANCER INCIDENCE

Cancer incidence and 5-year survival rates in Chapters 4–12 were derived from SEER registry data. The registries did not cover the entire United States, nor necessarily represent the entire population. Instead, each registry covers a specific set of counties, usually statewide, across diverse sections of the country. (For more information on registries, see SEER.[2, 3]) Population counts used for rates and age-adjustment were also restricted to the counties covered by the registry. Only estimates based on unweighted counts of 17 or more cases were shown, following the reporting standard set by NCI.

Cancer incidence was estimated for the entire country from the rates for the 17 registries in 2004, multiplied by the 2004 U.S. population. This yielded an estimated number of new cases for the United States in 2004. The unadjusted and age-adjusted incidence rates were based only on the 17 registry areas. Unadjusted rates were calculated from the number of new cases in 2004 divided by the population in the demographic subgroup. Age-adjusted incidence rates were calculated from the age-specific rates within the demographic subgroup multiplied by the U.S. standard 2000 population as described in section IV. Age-Adjustment.

VI. FIGURES
MORBIDITY ESTIMATES

The figures showing trends in ambulatory care visits and hospital discharges for the period 1979–2004 used the all-listed diagnoses. The all-listed diagnoses were defined the same as for the tables. However, the data source for hospital discharges was the NHDS because HCUP NIS data were unavailable over the entire timeframe. Because of the smaller sample size for the ambulatory care surveys, estimates derived from NAMCS/NHAMCS files were 3-year averages, except for the 1992 estimates, which were averages of 1992 and 1993 data. This approach provided more stable estimates across time. The year 1992 was the starting point, because this was the first year of the NHAMCS. All rates were age-adjusted.

MORTALITY

The figures showing mortality data for the period 1979–2004 used the multiple cause-of-death data for each year. Because these were observed counts for the United States and not samples, they were not considered estimates. The age-adjusted mortality rates were shown for both underlying cause and underlying or other cause for the total population per year. The vertical line at 1999 represented the change from ICD-9 to ICD-10.

CANCER INCIDENCE AND 5-YEAR SURVIVAL

For digestive cancers (Chapters 4–12), the figures for age-adjusted cancer incidence and 5-year survival were derived from data obtained by the nine registries that SEER used through the entire period 1979–2004. Five-year survival was the proportion of those diagnosed in a given year who were still known to be alive 5 years later. Five-year survival ended at 1999, because it was impossible to know the 5-year status of patients diagnosed after that year. Absolute survival is shown in these figures, whereas SEER typically publishes relative survival. Relative survival takes into account the expected survival of the population as a whole and is higher than absolute survival, especially for cancers that concentrate in groups with high underlying mortality, such as the elderly.

[1] Anderson RN, Rosenberg HM. Age standardization of death rates: implementation of the year 2000 standard. 3:1-20. October 7, 1998. *National Vital Statistics Reports*. Hyattsville Maryland: National Center for Health Statistics.

[2] *Surveillance, Epidemiology, and End Results (SEER) Program Limited-Use Data (1973–2005)* (www.seer.cancer.gov). National Cancer Institute, DCCPS, Surveillance Research Program, Cancer Statistics Branch. Released April 2008, based on the November 2007 submission.

[3] *US Population Data 1969–2005*. Downloaded from *SEER Program Populations (1969–2005)* (www.seer.cancer.gov/popdata). National Cancer Institute, DCCPS, Surveillance Research Program, Cancer Statistics Branch. Released April 2008.

Index of Tables and Figures

4.   Digestive Cancers

5.   Cancer of the Esophagus

6. Cancer of the Stomach

7. Cancer of the Small Intestine

11. Cancer of the Gallbladder

12. Cancer of the Pancreas

13. Hemorrhoids

14. Gastroesophageal Reflux Disease

15. Peptic Ulcer Disease

16. Functional Intestinal Disorders

17. Appendicitis

18. Abdominal Wall Hernia

19. Inflammatory Bowel Disease

20. Diverticular Disease

21. Liver Disease

22. Gallstones

23. Pancreatitis

24. Indications and Outcomes of Gastrointestinal Endoscopy

25. Costs of Digestive Diseases

Appendix 1. ICD and SEER Codes

www.ingramcontent.com/pod-product-compliance
Lightning Source LLC
Chambersburg PA
CBHW080411290526
45791CB00008BA/2229

* 9 7 8 1 4 9 4 8 5 3 0 3 7 *